FIRST AID

FIRST ON THE SCENE

EMERGENCY LEVEL

ACTIVITY BOOK

SECOND EDITION 1996

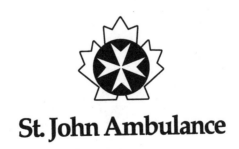

St. John Ambulance

First Edition - 1994
Second Edition - 1996
First Impression 1997 - 75,000
Second Impression 1998 - 75,000

St. John Ambulance
312 Laurier Avenue East
Ottawa, Ontario
K1N 6P6

Canadian Cataloguing in Publication Data

Main entry under title:

    First aid : first on the scene : emergency level : activity book

Includes index
ISBN 0-929006-74-7
(ISBN 0-929006-61-5. 1ˢᵗ edition, 1994)

    1. First aid in illness and injury. 2. CPR (First aid). 3. First aid in illness and injury—Problems, exercises, etc. 4. CPR (First aid)—Problems, exercises, etc. I. St. John Ambulance.

RC86.8.F593 1996   616.02'52   C96-900095-2

EpiPen® Auto Injector is a registered trademark of the EM Industries, Inc.
Ana-Kit® is a registered trademark of Miles Allergy Products Ltd.
Tylenol® is a registered trademark of McNeil Consumer Products.
Tempra® is a registered trademark of Mead Johnson Canada.

Cover design: Beth Haliburton
Cover photograph: Richard Desmarais
Cover art direction: David Craib
Illustrations: Stanley Berneche

Printed in Canada
Stock No. 6502

CONTENTS

STUDENT INFORMATION

St. John Ambulance Emergency and Standard Level first aid courses are nationally standardized programmes. They are based on performance objectives and well defined training standards which are contained in the Instructor's Guide for these courses.

This **self-instruction activity book** is part of a sequenced training programme, consisting of videos, instructor-led practical and activity book exercises.

Certification requirements

The training standards specify the minimum requirements for certification. Courses may be expanded, if necessary, to include additional material required to meet local needs.

To receive a certificate in *First Aid—Emergency Level*, you must obtain:

◆ a satisfactory pass on the practical exercises, and

◆ a minimum mark of 70% on each section of the written examination

Your first aid certificate is valid for three years from the month the course was successfully completed.

Note: First aid skills, and CPR skills in particular, deteriorate very quickly unless they are practised regularly. Recertification every three years in first aid and annual retraining in CPR is recommended.

The Manual

First on the Scene, The Complete Guide to First Aid and CPR, first edition, is the reference manual for this course. You may use the manual:

◆ as supplementary reading during the course, if time permits, or

◆ as reference material after the course

USE OF THE ACTIVITY BOOK

Before starting your activity book exercises, you should have completed the Course Registration Form contained at the back of this activity book and have handed it to your instructor.

Welcome to the activity book exercises.

This self-instruction book will help you to learn the first aid theory for the *First Aid— Emergency Level* course and will prepare you for the final written examination. Your instructor will tell you which exercises to complete and when to do them.

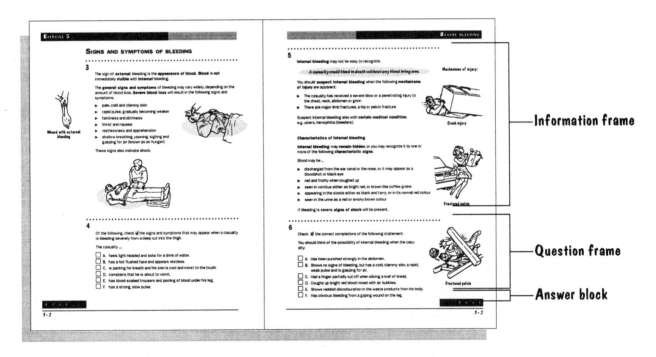

Each exercise consists of **teaching units** called **frames.**

Each frame is numbered and contains either:

◆ **information** for you to read, or

◆ **questions** for you to answer

The **correct answer** to each question appears in the **answer block** located at the bottom of the page.

How to do the activity book exercises

1. Tear off the **cursor** attached to the back cover.

2. Use the cursor to cover the answer block until you have marked your answers to the question.

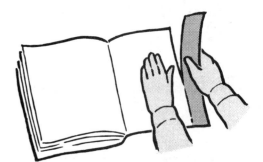

3. To **check** your answers, **slide the cursor to the side** as far as the end of the answer block. This will **reveal the correct** answer(s) in the answer block.

4. If your answer is wrong, read the question again, draw a line through your wrong answer and write in the correct one.

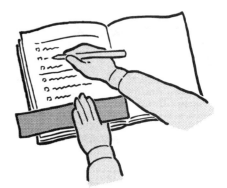

5. If you do not know the answer to a question, look at the answer frame, mark the correct answer in the appropriate space and read the question again.

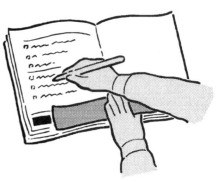

There are several types of questions used in this activity book to reinforce your learning. Four examples are given below:

Multiple choice type:

Check ☑ the correct completion to the statement below.

The aim of first aid for a minor, open wound is to:

- ☐ A. Prevent itching.
- ☐ B. Send the casualty to medical help.
- ☐ C. Control bleeding and prevent infection.
- ☐ D. Check the area around the wound.

Note: Multiple choice questions may have more than one right answer.

C

True or false type:

Mark each of the following statements as true **(T)** or false **(F)**:

☐ A. Spurting blood is more difficult to stop than flowing blood.
☐ B. Bleeding always looks the same, no matter where it comes from.

A.T B.F

Order type:

Number the following first aid actions in the order you should perform them:

☐ A. Send for medical help.
☐ B. Assess responsiveness.

A.2 B.1

Match type:

Match each situation with the appropriate safety measure.

Situations	Safety measures
☐ A. A girl gulps down a soft drink while chewing on her hamburger.	1. Avoid other activities when you are eating.
☐ B. A man eats a sandwich while trying to steer his car.	2. Don't eat and drink at the same time.

A.2 B.1

Instructor-led exercises:

The Instructor-led exercises will give you the opportunity to discuss and develop key ideas with the help of your instructor. To fill in the blanks properly, your instructor will give you the appropriate information. Should you do your activity book exercises at home, the answers to the instructor-led exercises are contained in Addendum C.

Instructor-led Exercise

A. Good air exchange	B. Poor air exchange	C. No air exchange
A1. The person _____ speak.	B1. The person _____ speak.	C1. The person _____ speak.
A2. The facial colour is	B2. The facial colour is	C2. The facial colour is
_____	_____	_____ .
A1. can	B1. cannot	C1. cannot
A2. reddish	B2. bluish	C2. bluish

EMERGENCY SCENE MANAGEMENT

Introduction to first aid

1

What is first aid?

First aid is the emergency help given to an injured or suddenly ill person using readily available materials.

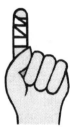

First aid symbol

The objectives of first aid **are to:**

◆ preserve life
◆ prevent the injury or illness from becoming worse
◆ promote recovery

Who is a first aider?

A first aider is someone who takes charge of an emergency scene and gives first aid.

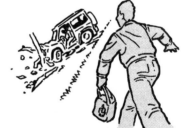

First aider arriving at the scene with a first aid kit

2

Mark each of the following statements as true **(T)** or false **(F)**.

☐ A. First aid is the immediate help you give to a person who is hurt or feels sick.

☐ B. You should never use anything except special dressings and bandages made for first aid.

☐ C. You may keep someone alive by giving first aid.

☐ D. Wounds have a better chance of healing if you give prompt and appropriate first aid.

☐ E. A first aider is a person who stops at a car crash and looks at the scene.

A.T B.F C.T D.T E.F

1-1

3

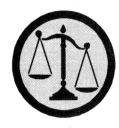

What can you do as a first aider?

You can help a person in need. Whenever you help a person in an emergency situation, you should abide by the **Principles of the Good Samaritan**, and:

◆ **act in good faith** and volunteer your help

◆ **tell the person you are a first aider**

◆ **get permission** (consent) to give first aid before touching the casualty. Use your common sense and consider the age and the condition of the casualty

◆ **ask** the parents or guardian for permission if the person is an infant or young child

◆ **have implied consent.** If the person does not **respond** to you, you can give first aid. Implied consent exists because the casualty is unconscious and does not object to your help

◆ **use reasonable skill and care** according to your level of knowledge and skills. Unless limited by a provincial statute, the care that is given to a person will be measured against what a reasonable person with similar knowledge and skills would do

◆ **do not abandon (leave) the person** once your offer of help has been accepted

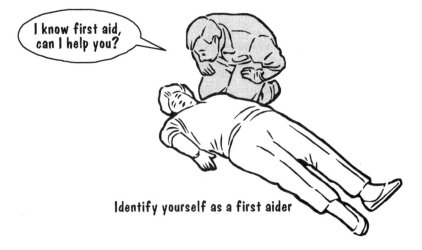

Identify yourself as a first aider

4

While walking in the park, you come across an elderly woman who has slipped on the ice. She is moaning in pain. What should you do? Check ☑ all correct answers below.

☑ A. Stop and see if you can help the person to feel better.

☑ B. You offer to help because you believe in good deeds.

☑ C. Immediately examine the person for any injuries.

☑ D. Introduce yourself as first aider and ask her to allow you to help.

☑ E. Give first aid to the best of your knowledge and ability.

☐ F. As soon as you have calmed down the lady, leave her alone.

5

What is medical help?

Medical help is the treatment given by, or under the supervision of, a medical doctor at an emergency scene, while transporting a casualty, or at a medical facility.

What is a casualty?

A person who is injured or who suddenly becomes ill is called a casualty.

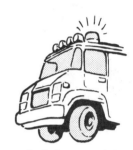

Doctor arriving on scene

Age guidelines for a casualty

For first aid and CPR techniques, a casualty is considered to be:

◆ **an adult** – eight years of age and over
◆ **a child** – from one to eight years of age
◆ **an infant** – under one year of age

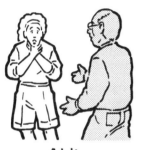

Adult

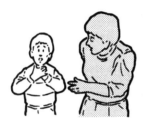

Child

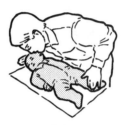

Infant

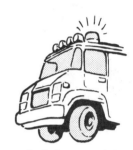

Ambulance arriving

Use these guidelines with **common sense** in choosing the appropriate first aid and CPR techniques. Consider the size of each casualty when making your decision.

Casualty with first aider

6

Mark each of the following statements as true **(T)** or false **(F)**.

[F] A. First aid is considered "medical help", if you have taken a first aid course.
[T] B. An ambulance attendant gives "medical help" because he works under the supervision of a doctor.
[T] C. A choking person who is unable to breathe is called a casualty.
[T] D. The term infant describes a baby who is less than one year old.
[F] E. A very small, delicate nine year-old should be treated as an adult when you give first aid.

A.F B.T C.T D.T E.F

Universal precautions in first aid

7

Some people are afraid to give first aid. They think they might catch a disease from the casualty. The risk of a serious infection being transmitted when giving first aid is small. Use the following **universal precautions** to minimize this risk and give first aid safely.

◆ **Wash your hands** with soap and running water immediately after any contact with a casualty

◆ **Wear vinyl or latex gloves** whenever you might be in touch with the casualty's blood, body fluids, open wounds or sores

◆ **Handle** sharp objects with extra care

◆ **Minimize** mouth-to-mouth contact during artificial respiration by using **a mask** or **a face shield** designed to prevent disease transmission

A face mask or face shield should:

◆ have a **one-way valve**

◆ be **disposable** or have a disposable valve

◆ be stored in an **easily accessible** place

Follow the manufacturer's instructions on how to use, care for and dispose of a mask and shield properly.

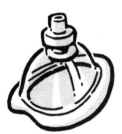

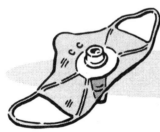

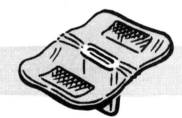

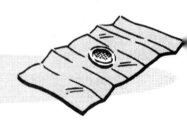

8

Which of the following actions should you take to protect yourself from infection when giving first aid?

Check ☑ your choice of answers.

☑ A. Avoid touching or being splashed by a casualty's blood or body fluids.

☑ B. Place an effective barrier between you and the casualty's body fluids.

☐ C. Don't give help to people you don't know.

☑ D. Keep from pricking yourself when touching needles or other sharp things.

☑ E. Be prepared with a first aid kit that includes disposable gloves and a face mask/shield.

How to remove gloves

. . . .

9

Gloves that have been used are contaminated and may spread infection. Take them off without touching the outside. Follow the steps below:

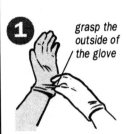

grasp the outside of the glove

Grasp the cuff of one glove.

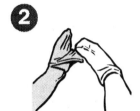

Pull the cuff towards the fingers, turning the glove inside out.

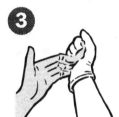

As the glove comes off, hold it in the palm of your other hand.

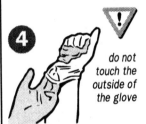

do not touch the outside of the glove

Slide your fingers under the cuff of the other glove.

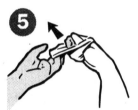

Pull the cuff towards the fingers over the first glove.

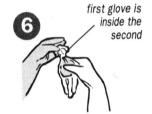

first glove is inside the second

Tie a knot in the top of the outer glove and dispose of properly—see below.

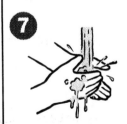

Wash hands with soap and running water as soon as possible.

Torn gloves

. . . .

If you tear your gloves while giving first aid, take them off right away. Wash your hands if possible, and put on a new pair of gloves.

Proper disposal

. . . .

Seal the used gloves in a plastic bag and put them in your household garbage.

Check with your instructor for specific regulations in your area.

Principles of emergency scene management (ESM)

10

Scene survey

Emergency scene management (ESM) is the sequence of actions you should follow at the scene of an emergency to ensure that safe and appropriate first aid is given.

The **ESM** has four steps:

◆ scene survey

◆ primary survey

◆ secondary survey (taught as an elective lesson 10). This step may not need to be done if first aid for life-threatening conditions has been given and medical help is on the way.

◆ ongoing casualty care until hand over

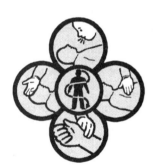

Primary survey

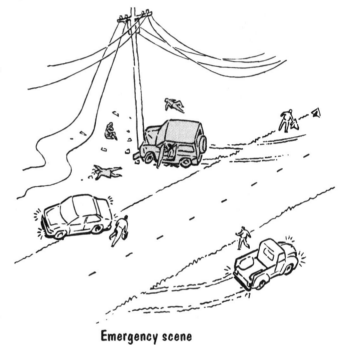

Emergency scene

Secondary survey

11

Ongoing casualty care

Of the following sentences, check ☑ the correct statements regarding emergency scene management.

☐ A. You should change the order of the steps of emergency scene management based on the type of injury or illness.

☑ B. Emergency scene management starts with the survey of the scene and ends when you have handed over the casualty to medical help.

☒ C. You have to do all four steps of emergency scene management every time you give first aid.

☑ D. Following the steps of emergency scene management will help you to give the best possible care to a casualty.

12

Scene survey

The order of steps in the scene survey may change, but in most cases, you will do them in this order:

- take charge of the situation. If head/spinal injuries are suspected, tell casualty not to move.

- call for help to attract bystanders

- assess hazards at the scene and make the area safe for yourself and others

- determine the number of casualties, what happened and the mechanism of injury for each

- identify yourself as a first aider. Offer to help and obtain consent.

- if head/spinal injuries are suspected, do not move the casualty. Provide and maintain manual support for the head and neck.

- assess the casualty's responsiveness. If the casualty is not responsive, send or go for medical help.

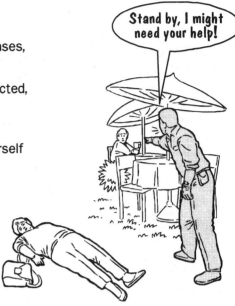

Stand by, I might need your help!

Scene survey

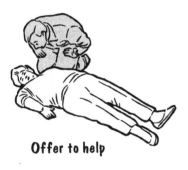

Offer to help

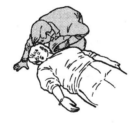

Assess responsiveness

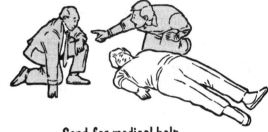

Send for medical help

13

Mark each of the following statements as true **(T)** or false **(F)**.

A. When approaching an emergency scene, the first thing you should do is take the lead and try to get someone to help.

B. At a car crash site, you give first aid without worrying about further dangers to yourself and the casualty.

C. To give appropriate first aid, you should check how many people are hurt and how badly.

D. Before you touch an injured person, you should introduce yourself and ask if you can help.

E. If you think that a casualty's neck has been hurt, tell him not to move. Steady his head and neck with your hands or show a bystander how to do this.

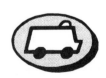

A.T B.F C.T D.T E.T

14

To help you to decide on the urgency of getting medical help, find out about the . . .

Scene survey

Number of casualties

◆ How many people were hurt

History (what, how, why)

◆ The full story of what happened
◆ How the injuries or illness happened
◆ The circumstances leading to or surrounding the incident

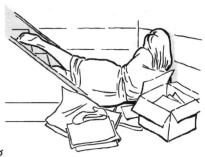

Casualty crumpled at the bottom of stairs

Mechanism of injury

◆ The force that causes the injury and the way it is applied to the body

Important information when you are assessing the mechanism of injury includes:

◆ the type of force
◆ the height of a fall
◆ the speed of a vehicle involved
◆ the location on the body

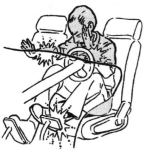

Body hits steering wheel

The greater the force, height or speed, the more likely it is that injuries will be life-threatening.

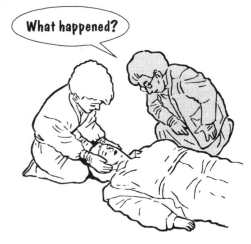

What happened?

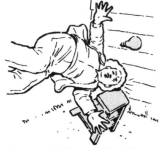

Worker falling off ladder

15

Place a check mark ☑ beside the described mechanisms of injury that are more likely to cause life-threatening injuries and would require fast medical help.

☑ A. A high speed car crash involving several people.
☐ B. Bumping into someone on the sidewalk.
☑ C. A person diving into a shallow pool and hitting his head.
☐ D. A heavy box falling on a person's foot.
☑ E. A truck crushing somebody against a wall.
☑ F. A person falling off the roof of a house.

A C E F

16

To help you decide what first aid to give to a casualty, you should find out as much as possible about the casualty's injury or illness. You need three kinds of information:

◆ history

◆ signs and

◆ symptoms

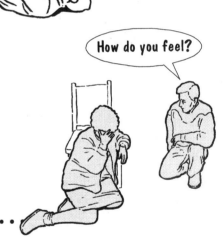

What happened?

History

◆ **Ask** the conscious casualty "what happened?"

◆ **Ask** bystanders "what happened?"

◆ **Observe** the scene

What do I see, hear, feel, smell?

Signs

Signs are conditions of the casualty **you can see, hear, feel or smell.**

◆ **Observe** the casualty

◆ **Examine** for indications of injury or illness

How do you feel?

Symptoms

Symptoms are **things the casualty feels** and may be able to describe.

◆ **Ask** the conscious casualty how she feels

◆ **Listen** to what the casualty says

17

Identify the information of each statement below as either history, sign or symptom by writing the appropriate number into the boxes provided.

History ☐1 Sign ☐2 Symptom ☐3

3 A. A casualty tells you he feels cold.

2 B. There is blood soaking through the shirt on a casualty's arm.

2 C. A casualty's skin is cold and clammy to the touch.

1 D. A man tells you that he slipped on a patch of ice.

3 E. A young boy says he feels sick.

1 F. You see an empty bottle of sleeping pills near an unconscious person.

A.3 B.2 C.2 D.1 E.3 F.1

Primary survey

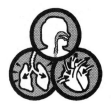

18

The primary survey is the first step in assessing the casualty for life-threatening conditions and giving life-saving first aid.

In the primary survey you check for the **priorities of first aid**. These are:

A. Airway – to ensure a clear airway

B. Breathing – to ensure effective breathing

C. Circulation – to ensure effective circulation

Even if there is more than one casualty, you should perform a primary survey on each casualty in turn. Give life-saving first aid only.

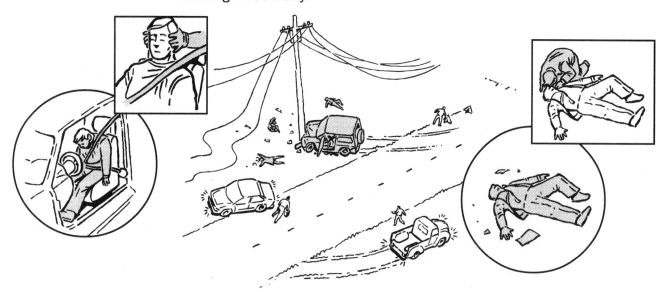

19

From the following statements, check ☑ all correct endings to the following two statements.

The purpose of the primary survey is to:

☑ A. Find all injuries.

☑ B. Find the conditions posing an immediate danger to life.

☐ C. Give complete treatment to all injuries.

Immediate threats to life include the following conditions:

☑ D. A blocked airway.

☑ E. Severe bleeding inside the body.

☐ F. A broken arm.

☑ G. Stopped breathing.

B D E G

Steps of the primary survey

. . . .

20

The sequential steps of the primary survey should be performed in **the position found**, unless it is impossible to do so.

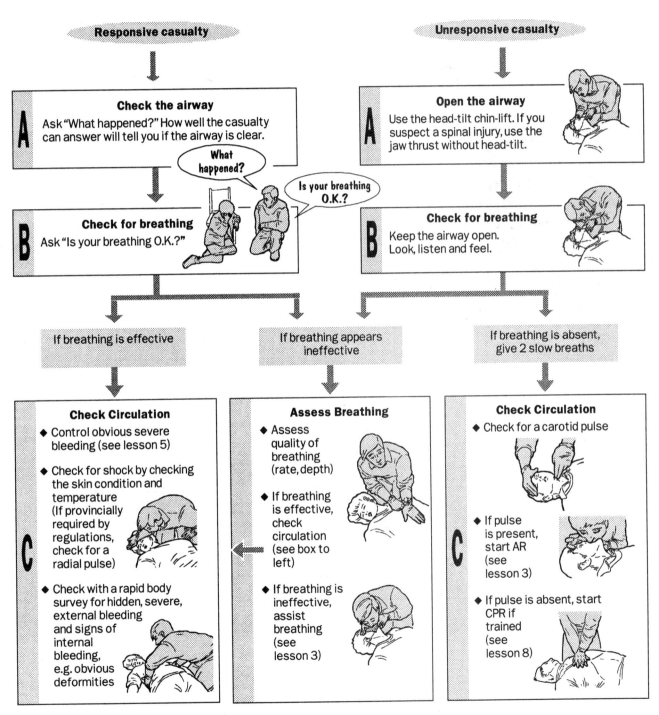

When you check the ABC's, give first aid as soon as you find any life-threatening condition.
If you find any deformities, manually steady and support the injured part until medical help takes over.

21

You have finished the scene survey. The mechanism of injury does not lead you to suspect a spinal injury. You know that the casualty is unresponsive. This means you have consent to help. You have to do the primary survey to find out if the casualty has any life-threatening injuries.

Keeping the priorities of first aid in mind, place these first aid actions in the **right sequence**. Write the appropriate number into the boxes provided.

A. Check breathing.

B. Check how the skin feels. Is it dry, wet, cool, warm?

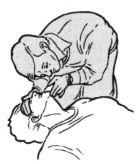

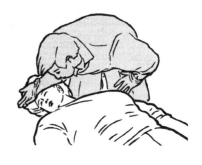

C. Open the airway.

D. Check quickly if the casualty has other life-threatening injuries.

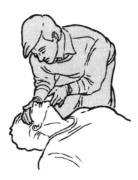

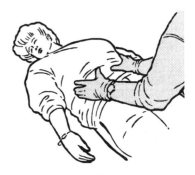

A.2 B.3 C.1 D.4

Ongoing casualty care until hand over

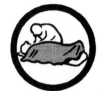

22

Following immediate first aid, you must **maintain the casualty in the best possible condition until hand over to medical help**.

- ◆ Instruct a bystander to maintain manual support of head and neck, if head/spinal injuries are suspected
- ◆ Continue to steady and support any injuries manually, if needed
- ◆ Give first aid for shock
  - ❖ reassure the casualty often
  - ❖ loosen tight clothing
  - ❖ place the casualty in the best position for her injury or illness
  - ❖ cover the casualty to preserve body heat
- ◆ Monitor the casualty's condition (ABC's) and note any changes
- ◆ Give nothing by mouth
- ◆ Record the casualty's condition, any changes that may occur and the first aid given
- ◆ Protect the casualty's personal belongings
- ◆ Do not leave the casualty until medical help takes over
- ◆ Hand over to medical help and report on the incident, the casualty's condition and the first aid given

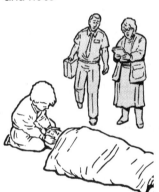

Shock position

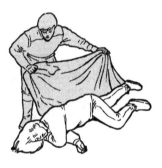

Supporting head and neck

Recovery position

23

An ambulance is expected soon.

Which of the actions listed below should you take to care for a conscious casualty following immediate first aid? Check off ☑ your choices.

- ☑ A. Place a blanket under and over the casualty to maintain body temperature.
- ☑ B. Check skin temperature and condition frequently.
- ☑ C. Provide hand support to injured body parts.
- ☐ D. Leave the casualty alone without further checking.
- ☑ E. Report to medical personnel on the casualty's condition and the help given.
- ☑ F. Make sure that the casualty doesn't lose any valuables.

A B C   E F

Objectives

- -

Following the videos and upon completion of your practical skills and this activity book exercise, in an emergency situation, you will be able to:

◆ apply the knowledge of terms used in first aid

◆ apply the knowledge of legal implications when giving first aid

◆ apply the principles of safety when giving first aid

◆ apply the principles of first aid

◆ apply the principles of emergency scene management

◆ perform a scene survey

◆ perform a primary survey

◆ perform ongoing casualty care until hand over

◆ perform the sequential steps of emergency scene management

For further information on emergency scene management, please refer to:
First on the Scene, the St. John Ambulance first aid and CPR manual, chapter 1 and 2, available through your instructor or any major bookstore in your area.

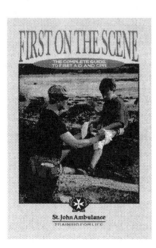

SHOCK, UNCONSCIOUSNESS AND FAINTING

1

Shock is a condition of **inadequate circulation** to the body tissues. It results when the brain and other vital organs are deprived of oxygen. The development of shock can **be gradual or rapid.**

Shock may be present with most injuries and illnesses.

Common causes of severe shock	
Cause of shock	**How it affects the circulation**
◆ breathing problems (ineffective or absent breathing)	not enough oxygen in the blood to supply the vital organs
◆ severe bleeding, external or internal, including major fractures	not enough blood in circulation to supply all vital organs
◆ severe burns	loss of fluids, reducing amount of blood to fill the blood vessels
◆ spinal cord injuries	nervous system can't control the size of blood vessels and blood pools away from vital organs
◆ heart attack	heart is not strong enough to pump blood properly
◆ medical emergencies, e.g. diabetes, allergies, poisoning	these conditions may affect breathing, heart and nerve function

Shock can be life

threatening and needs

to be recognized and

cared for immediately.

2

Of the following sentences, check ☑ each true statement.

     A. Shock occurs when vital body parts do not receive enough blood.

     B. A casualty with severe bleeding will show signs of shock.

     C. Shock is caused only by life-threatening injuries.

     D. A casualty always shows signs of shock right after the injury occurs.

     E. Shock may become life-threatening.

A B E

Signs and symptoms of shock

. . . .

3

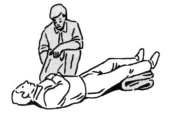

The **signs** and **symptoms** of shock may not be obvious immediately, but any of the following may appear as shock progresses.

You may see:

- restlessness
- decreased consciousness
- pale skin at first, later bluish grey
- bluish/purple colour to lips, tongue, earlobes and fingernails*
- cold, clammy skin
- profuse sweating
- vomiting
- shallow, irregular breathing; could be rapid and gasping for air
- a weak, rapid pulse (in later stages the radial pulse may be absent)

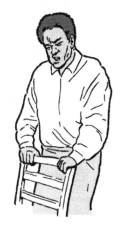

* **Note:** If the casualty has dark skin, the inside of the lips, the mouth, the tongue and the nail beds will be blue; the skin around the nose and mouth greyish.

The casualty may tell you of:

- feelings of anxiety and doom
- being confused and dizzy
- extreme thirst
- nausea
- faintness
- pain

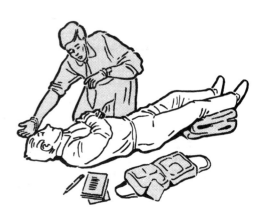

Check skin condition

. . . .

4

From the choices below, check ☑ the correct completion for the following statement. Write the appropriate choice number into the boxes provided:

	When a casualty is in shock, usually the . . .	Choice 1	Choice 2
1	A. skin is	white	reddish
2	B. skin is	dry	moist
2	C. skin is	warm	cold
1	D. breathing is	fast	slow
1	E. pulse is	fast	slow
2	F. casualty feels	calm	uneasy
1	G. casualty feels	thirsty	hungry

First aid for shock

. . . .

5

To prevent shock from becoming worse:

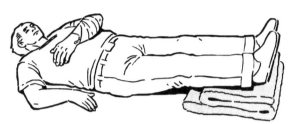

◆ **give prompt and effective first aid for any injury or illness**

◆ reassure the casualty often

◆ loosen tight clothing at neck, chest and waist

◆ place the casualty into the best position for the condition

◆ cover the casualty to preserve body heat

◆ place a blanket under the casualty, if available. Ensure movement does not aggravate injuries

◆ give nothing by mouth

◆ moisten lips only if the casualty complains of thirst

◆ monitor the casualty's condition (ABC's) and note any changes

◆ continue ongoing casualty care until hand over to medical help

Shock position
feet and legs raised
about 30 cm (12 inches)

Conscious casualty

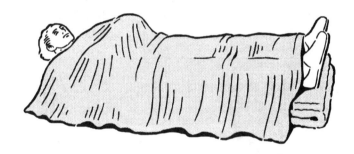

Covered casualty in shock position

. . . .

6

A conscious casualty is bleeding from a large slash on his forearm. His skin is cold and moist. His lips and earlobes appear bluish. Of the following, check ☑ the first aid actions you should take to prevent the casualty's condition from becoming worse.

☑ A. Give immediate first aid for the wound.

☐ B. Place the casualty into the recovery position.

☑ C. Place covers under and over the casualty to keep him warm.

☐ D. Give the casualty water to drink since he is complaining of severe thirst.

☐ E. Rub the casualty's limbs vigorously to improve his circulation.

☑ F. Avoid causing the casualty more discomfort.

A · C · F

Positioning of a casualty in shock

7

The **position** you use for a casualty **depends on the casualty's condition.**
Always consider the casualty's comfort when choosing a position.

◆ To prevent further injury, support a casualty with suspected head/spinal injuries in the:

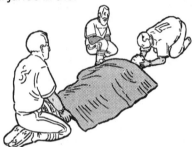

Position found

◆ To ease breathing, place a casualty with breathing difficulty, e.g. heart attack, asthma, into the:

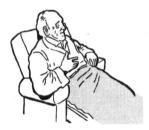

Semisitting position

◆ To maintain an open airway, place the unresponsive casualty into the:

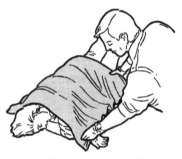

Recovery position

◆ To increase blood flow to the vital organs, place the conscious casualty into the:

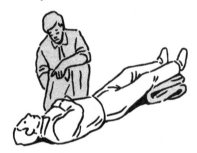

Shock position

8

Match the condition of each casualty with the position you would use to prevent shock and aggravation of injury. Place the appropriate number in the boxes provided.

Condition	Position
[3] A. Possible neck injury.	1. Recovery position
[1] B. Unresponsive but breathing.	2. Semisitting position
[4] C. A conscious casualty's leg is bleeding severely.	3. Position found
[2] D. Breathing difficulty due to chest pain.	4. Shock position

A.3 B.1 C.4 D.2

First aid for shock—review

9

The following question is based on the video, your practical exercise and this activity book exercise.

Your friend is working alone in a wood workshop. The chain saw slips and causes a large slash in your friend's lower arm. The cut is bleeding profusely and your friend is pale and sweating as you arrive.

What sequence of actions would you follow at this emergency scene to give appropriate first aid and slow down the progress of shock?

 A. Check the airway by asking: "Where do you hurt?"

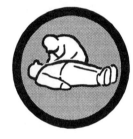

 B. Expose the wound and control severe bleeding.

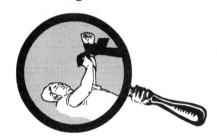

C. Survey the scene.

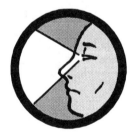

 D. Check breathing by asking: "Is your breathing O.K.?"

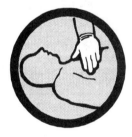

E. Give ongoing casualty care.

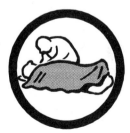

 F. Check the skin condition and temperature; and perform a rapid body survey.

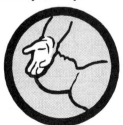

A.2 B.4 C.1 D.3 E.6 F.5

Unconsciousness

. . . .

10

When you assess a casualty and find her unresponsive, you should immediately:

◆ send, or go for medical help

If the casualty remains unresponsive, she is considered to be unconscious.

Unconsciousness indicates a serious medical situation. Many injuries and illnesses are complicated by the loss of consciousness, e.g. head injuries, breathing emergencies, heart attack, poisoning, shock and fainting.

Unconsciousness is a *breathing emergency*.

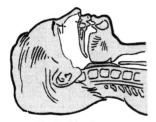

Tongue blocking
the airway

If the unconscious casualty is lying on his back, the airway may become blocked by the tongue falling to the back of the throat, or by fluids draining into the airway. Maintaining effective breathing is the *first priority*.

◆ Look, listen and feel to determine if the casualty is breathing

◆ **Recheck breathing** frequently

◆ If the casualty stops breathing, give artificial respiration immediately.

Fluids blocking
the airway

First aid for an *unconscious* casualty (when medical help is on the way)

◆ Perform a primary survey
◆ Give first aid for any life-threatening conditions
◆ Loosen restrictive clothing
◆ Place the casualty into the recovery position, if injuries permit
◆ Give ongoing casualty care until hand over to medical help

Any change in the casualty's condition should be observed and noted, and described to medical personnel when the casualty is handed over.

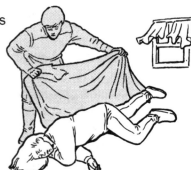

Recovery position

. . . .

11

A woman collapses in the shopping mall. When you call out to her and tap her on the shoulders, you determine that she is unresponsive (unconscious). Order the following actions according to your priorities by placing the appropriate number into the squares provided:

1 A. Ask a bystander to telephone for an ambulance.

3 B. Apply first aid for life-threatening conditions.

4 C. Loosen the casualty's collar and belt.

2 D. Perform a primary survey.

5 E. Place the casualty in the recovery position, if injuries permit.

Fainting

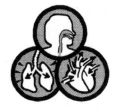

12

Fainting is a brief loss of consciousness caused by a **temporary shortage of oxygen to the brain.**

Fainting may be caused by:

◆ fatigue, hunger or lack of fresh air

◆ fear and anxiety

◆ long periods of standing or sitting

◆ severe pain, injury or illness

The following may warn you that a person is about to faint:

◆ you may observe paleness and sweating

◆ the casualty may complain of feeling sick and dizzy

Shock position

 First aid for the person who feels fainted

Act quickly (you may be able to prevent her from fainting):

◆ lay the person down with legs raised about 30 cm (12 in) (shock position)

◆ ensure a supply of fresh air

◆ loosen tight clothing around the neck, chest and waist

If you cannot lay the person down:

◆ have the person sit with the head and shoulders lowered

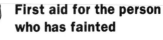 **First aid for the person who has fainted**

A person who has fainted is temporarily unconscious. The first aid is the same as for the person who is unconscious (see opposite page).

When the casualty regains consciousness:

◆ make her comfortable

◆ keep her lying down for 10 to 15 minutes

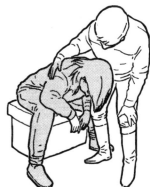

Sitting position

13

When a person in a small, overcrowded meeting room turns pale, and says that she feels sick and unsteady, what should you do? Check ☑ the correct answers.

☑ A. Open the windows or door.

☐ B. Tilt her head back and press a cold towel on her forehead.

☑ C. Unbutton her shirt at the neck and loosen her belt.

☑ D. Place her at rest on the back and put a rolled-up jacket under her ankles.

☐ E. Obtain medical help immediately.

A   C   D

Objectives

• •

Following the video and upon completion of your practical skills and this activity book exercise, in an emergency situation, you will be able to:

◆ recognize shock
◆ provide first aid for shock
◆ recognize unconsciousness
◆ provide first aid for unconsciousness
◆ recognize fainting
◆ provide first aid for fainting

For further information on first aid for shock, unconsciousness and fainting, please refer to: *First on the Scene*, the St. John Ambulance first aid and CPR manual, chapter 1, available through your instructor or any major bookstore in your area.

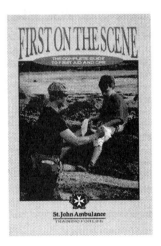

ARTIFICIAL RESPIRATION–ADULT

Introduction to breathing emergencies

1

We must breathe to live!

Breathing is the movement of air in and out of the lungs.

Air is taken in and out of the lungs by **the respiratory system** which has three main parts:

◆ the airway

◆ the lungs and

◆ the diaphragm

Air reaches our lungs through the **airway**.

Respiration is the process of exchange of oxygen (O_2) and carbon dioxide (CO_2) in the body.

◆ The air we breathe in contains **oxygen,** which is important to life

◆ The air we breathe out contains **carbon dioxide**, a waste product of the body

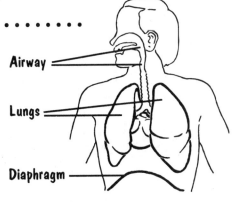

Airway

Lungs

Diaphragm

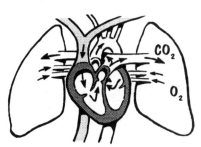

Gas Exchange

2

Check ☑ the correct statements below:

☑ A. The airway is the passage through which air flows to get from the nose and mouth to the lungs.

☑ B. The function of breathing allows air to pass in and out of the lungs.

☐ C. Carbon dioxide is the most important part of the air we breathe in.

☑ D. Our bodies need a frequent new supply of oxygen to survive.

A B D

Causes of breathing emergencies

3

The causes of breathing emergencies can be classified into **three major groups:**

◆ there is not enough oxygen in the air
◆ the heart and lungs are not working properly
◆ the airway is blocked—the person is choking

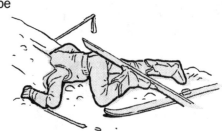

Life-threatening breathing emergencies can result from:

◆ suffocation
◆ airway obstruction
◆ head/spinal injuries
◆ electric shock
◆ drug overdose

◆ heart attack
◆ near-drowning
◆ open chest wound
◆ poisoning
◆ allergic reactions, e.g. asthma

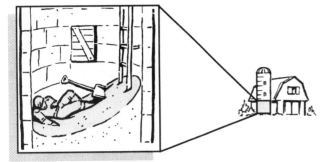

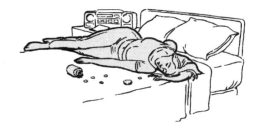

4

Check ☑ the correct completions to the following statements. Breathing emergencies occur when:

A. a person is deprived of ...

☐ 1. carbon dioxide in inhaled air.
☑ 2. oxygen in inhaled air.

B. air is not reaching a person's lungs because of a blocked ...

☐ 1. nasal passage.
☑ 2. airway.

C. a person has poor functioning of the ...

☑ 1. respiratory system.
☐ 2. muscles in the body.

Signs of breathing emergencies

5

When breathing **stops** or is **ineffective**, the body is deprived of oxygen. This is called a breathing emergency.

After **4 minutes** without oxygen, brain damage may result.

You must act immediately to restore breathing or assist breathing!

Be alert for signs of breathing emergencies:

Breathing has **stopped**, when . . .

◆ the chest does not rise and fall
◆ air movement cannot be heard or felt

Ineffective breathing is generally characterized by . . .

◆ very slow and shallow breaths, 10 or less per minute
◆ very fast and shallow breaths, about 30 or more per minute
◆ laboured and noisy breathing, gasping for air
◆ sweaty skin
◆ fatigue
◆ a bluish colour to the skin
◆ decreased level of consciousness

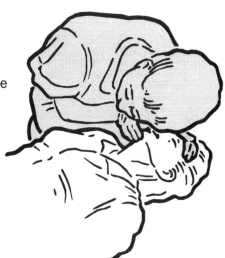
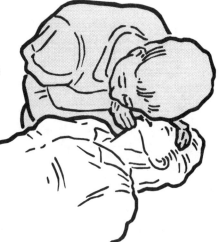

Check for breathing

6

From the following statements, check ☑ the signs which may indicate a breathing emergency:

◻ A. The chest expands and relaxes with ease.
☑ B. Rapid, irregular chest movement.
☑ C. No chest movement when you watch for breathing.
◻ D. Regular and quiet breaths.
☑ E. A casualty's lips and earlobes show blue discolouration.
☑ F. A great effort needed to breathe, making the casualty very tired.

B C E F

Effective breathing

7

Effective breathing usually is . . .

◆ without pain or effort
◆ easy and quiet
◆ with even steady rhythm

To check the **effectiveness** of the casualty's breathing, you assess the . . .

◆ breathing rate
◆ breathing depth and quality
◆ skin colour

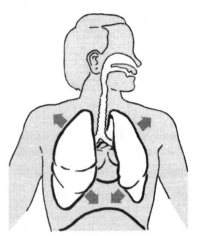

**Breathing in—
lungs inflate**

Breathing rate

◆ Is the number of breaths in one minute
◆ The average breathing rate for a healthy adult at rest is in the range of
  10 to 20 breaths per minute

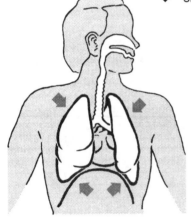

**Breathing out—
lungs deflate**

8

Mark each statement below as true **(T)** or false **(F)**:

A. A person having 14 breaths a minute fits within the normal range of breathing.

B. Breathing in and breathing out should be smooth and painless.

C. A casualty's breathing is adequate, when you observe deep, sucking breaths.

D. If you suspect that a casualty's breathing is ineffective, count the number of breaths per minute and check the skin colour.

E. You should immediately try to breathe for a person who shows no signs of air moving in or out of the lungs.

A.T B.T C.F D.T E.T

First aid for breathing emergencies

9

When breathing stops, a person requires **immediate first aid**.

◆ You must get oxygen into the casualty's lungs

◆ The oxygen content of the air you breathe out is **enough to sustain** the life of a non-breathing person. The best way to do this is by blowing into the casualty's mouth. This is called **mouth-to-mouth artificial respiration (AR)**

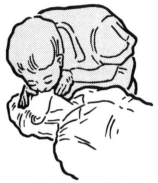

Mouth-to-mouth AR

Blowing into the casualty's nose is another method of AR, the **mouth-to-nose method of AR**.

◆ Use the mouth-to-nose method when . . .

  ◆ the mouth cannot be opened

  ◆ the casualty has injuries about the mouth or jaw

  ◆ your mouth cannot fully cover the casualty's mouth

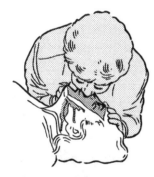

**Mouth-to-nose AR
with shield**

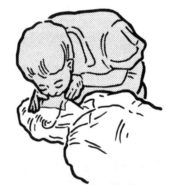

**Mouth-to-mouth AR
with shield**

10

From the listing below, check ☑ the correct statements relating to first aid for a non-breathing casualty.

☑ A. You can keep a person alive by blowing into her mouth or nose.

☑ B. The mouth-to-mouth method of AR is the best way you can get air into the casualty's lungs.

☐ C. If a casualty has a broken chin, use the mouth-to-mouth method of AR.

A   B

Mouth-to-nose method of AR

· ·

11

The basic techniques for the mouth-to-nose method are the same as for the mouth-to-mouth, **except that you breathe through the casualty's nose.**

The mouth-to-mouth method is modified for the mouth-to-nose method by the following techniques:

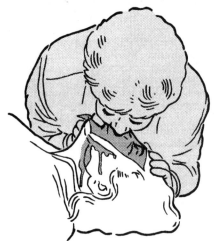

Mouth-to-nose

- ◆ **tilt** the head back using the head-tilt chin-lift
- ◆ **close** the casualty's mouth with your thumb
- ◆ **cover** the casualty's nose with your mouth to give ventilations
- ◆ **give a ventilation and watch** the chest rise
- ◆ **open** the casualty's mouth between breaths and remove your mouth from the casualty's nose to let the air out
- ◆ **look, listen** and **feel** for air movement

· ·

12

Check ☑ the correct completions for the following statement. When using the mouth-to-nose method of artificial respiration, you . . .

A. blow air into the casualty's . . .

  ☐ 1. mouth.
  ☑ 2. nose.

B. prevent air leakage by using your thumb to close the . . .

  ☑ 1. mouth.
  ☐ 2. nose.

C. allow air to escape between breaths by opening the . . .

  ☑ 1. mouth.
  ☐ 2. nose.

A.2 B.1 C.1

Assisted breathing

13

You may have to assist a casualty to breathe if he has severe breathing difficulties.

The **responsive** casualty may resist your efforts to assist breathing.

◆ **Reassure** the casualty and **explain** what you are trying to do and why it is needed

◆ Do not attempt to assist breathing if the casualty remains uncooperative

The **unresponsive** casualty with ineffective breathing ...

◆ is in urgent need of your assistance

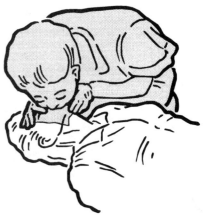

**Mouth-to-mouth with shield
(head-tilt chin-lift)**

How to provide assisted breathing

The technique for assisted breathing is the same as for mouth-to-mouth AR, except for the timing of the ventilations.

If the breathing rate is below 10 breaths per minute ...

◆ match the casualty's inhalations. Give additional ventilations between the casualty's own breaths to a combined total of 1 breath every 5 seconds

If the breathing rate is greater than 30 breaths per minute ...

◆ assist every second breath to slow the casualty's breathing rate. This will result in more effective breathing

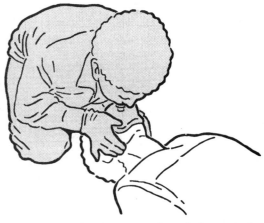

**Mouth-to-mouth with face mask
(jaw-thrust)**

14

From the options below, check ☑ the correct completion to the following statement:

You should provide assisted breathing for severe respiratory distress when the casualty is:

☑ A. Breathing less than 10 times per minute.

☐ B. Conscious and refusing your help to assist him in his breathing.

☑ C. Breathing 35 times per minute.

☐ D. Unconscious, breathing quietly and has a good skin colour.

A C

Gastric distension and vomiting during AR

. . . .

15

Gastric distension and **vomiting** during AR are usually caused by **increased air in the stomach.** This happens when...

◆ the airway is not completely open

◆ ventilations are given too quickly and with too much force causing air to enter the stomach. This prevents effective ventilation

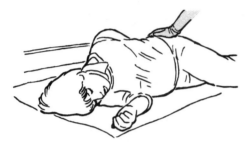

Gastric distension

To reduce the risk of gastric distension:

◆ ensure an open airway

◆ give slow breaths

◆ use only enough air to make the chest rise

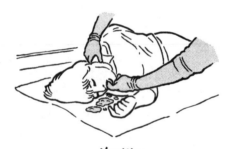

Vomiting

If vomiting occurs during AR:

◆ turn the casualty to the side with her head turned down

◆ wipe the mouth clear of vomitus

◆ reposition the casualty on her back

◆ reassess breathing and pulse

◆ resume ventilations

. . . .

16

Check ☑ the correct procedures that should be followed...

A. to lessen the possibility of air getting into the casualty's stomach:

    ☑ 1. recheck and maintain an open airway.

    ☑ 2. avoid breathing too fast and too strongly into the casualty.

B. when vomiting occurs:

    ☑ 1. position the casualty for good drainage. Clear her mouth, check breathing and pulse and continue AR.

    ☐ 2. rinse the casualty's mouth thoroughly after clearing.

Artificial respiration—review

· ·

17

The following questions are based on the videos, your practical exercises and this activity book exercise.

You witness a near-drowning on a beach with a few bystanders standing around the casualty. It wasn't a diving incident and there is no indication of head/spinal injuries. You take charge and begin emergency scene management.

Number the following first aid actions for this casualty **in the order you should perform them.** Place the appropriate numbers in the squares provided.

6 A. Check for a carotid pulse.

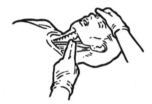

3 B. Open the airway.

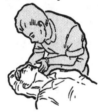

1 C. Assess responsiveness.

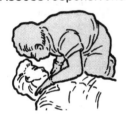

5 D. Give two slow breaths.

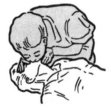

7 E. Continue giving one breath every five seconds.

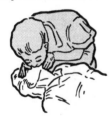

4 F. Check for breathing.

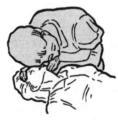

2 G. Send a bystander to get medical help.

Get medical help!

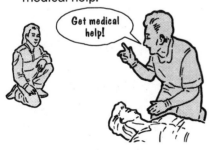

A.6 B.3 C.1 D.5 E.7 F.4 G.2

Objectives

· ·

Following the video and upon completion of your practical skills and this activity book exercise, in an emergency situation, you will be able to:

◆ apply the basic knowledge of the respiratory system

◆ recognize breathing emergencies

◆ perform mouth-to-mouth artificial respiration (AR) on an adult casualty

◆ perform mouth-to-mouth AR on an adult casualty with suspected head/spinal injuries

◆ perform mouth-to-nose AR on an adult casualty

◆ deal with two complications that may occur when giving AR

◆ provide assisted breathing

For further information on first aid for breathing emergencies, please refer to: *First on the Scene*, the St. John Ambulance first aid and CPR manual, chapter 4, available through your instructor or any major bookstore in your area.

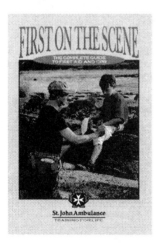

CHOKING–ADULT

Signs of choking and first aid

1

A person chokes when the airway is partly or completely blocked and airflow is reduced or cut off. A choking person may die if first aid is not given **immediately**.

A person's airway can be either: **partially** or **completely** blocked.

A **partially** blocked airway results in either:

◆ **good air exchange**

◆ **poor air exchange**

With a **completely** blocked airway, there is:

◆ **no air exchange**

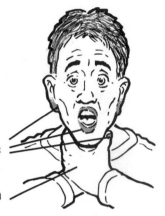

discolouration of lips, earlobes and fingernails

universal sign of choking

2 Instructor-led Exercise 4

A. Good air exchange	**B. Poor air exchange**	**C. No air exchange**
A1. The person _Can_ speak.	B1. The person _Can't_ speak.	C1. The person _Cant_ speak.
A2. Coughing and gagging are _forceful_.	B2. Coughing and gagging are _ineffective_.	C2. Coughing and gagging are _Impossible_.
A3. You may hear _wheezing_ when trying to breathe.	B3. You may hear _high pitched Sound_ when trying to breathe.	C3. There will be _no Sound_; the person _can't breath_ breathe.
A4. The facial colour is _Red_.	B4. The facial colour is _blueish_.	C4. The facial colour is _blue_.
A5. Stand by and _encourage_	B5. Start _first aid_ for choking.	C5. Start _first aid_ for choking.

Answers: Addendum C

Causes and prevention of choking

. . . .

3

Choking is a life-threatening **breathing emergency.** A choking person may die if first aid for choking is not given **immediately.**

Common causes of choking are:

◆ food or some other object stuck in the throat

◆ the tongue of an unconscious person falling to the back of the throat

◆ blood or vomit collects in the throat

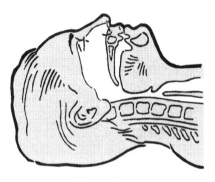

Clear airway

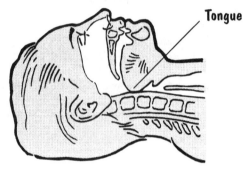

Tongue

Blocked airway by tongue

. . . .

4

Check ☑ the correct answers from either choice 1 or choice 2 to complete the following statements.

| Choice 1 | Choice 2 |

When a casualty is choking and has poor or no air exchange . . .

☐ A. the air passages are clear.	☑ A. the air passages are blocked.
☑ B. there is little or no air getting to the lungs.	☐ B. air flows freely into and out of the lungs.
☑ C. his life is in danger.	☐ C. his life is not in danger.

When a casualty is unconscious . . .

| ☐ D. his air passages open wider. | ☑ D. his tongue may block the air passages. |

A.2 B.1 C.1 D.2

5

Choking may be caused by:

◆ trying to swallow large pieces of food
◆ eating and drinking while doing something else
◆ drinking too much alcohol before or during a meal
◆ gulping drinks with food in your mouth

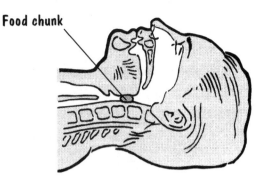

Airway blocked by food chunk

Avoid choking by taking these precautions:

◆ chew food well before swallowing
◆ avoid talking and laughing while chewing food
◆ drink alcohol in moderation before and during meals
◆ avoid other physical activities while eating

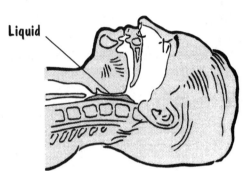

Airway partially blocked by liquid

6

Listed below are dangerous situations that could cause choking.

Match each situation with the appropriate safety measure. Place the correct number in the boxes provided.

Situations	**Safety measures**
A. A teenager shoves a hot dog into his mouth and gulps it down quickly.	1. Don't eat and drink at the same time.
B. A man eats a sandwich while driving his car.	2. Cut food into small pieces and chew it well before you swallow.
C. A girl gulps down a soft drink while chewing on her hamburger.	3. Avoid other activities when you are eating.
	4. Cut food lengthwise so it won't get caught in the throat.

A.2 B.3 C.1

Self-administered first aid for choking

7

Abdominal thrusts

When you are alone and choke and **you cannot speak, breathe or cough,** you can help yourself.

◆ Try to call for medical help (call 911 if available in your area) or to attract attention

Using your hands:

◆ place a fist above your navel
◆ grasp the fist with the other hand
◆ press inward and upward forcefully. Make each thrust distinct, with the intent to dislodge the obstruction
◆ repeat thrusts until the obstruction is relieved

Using furniture:

◆ position your abdominal area, slightly above the hips, along the counter, table edge or the back of a chair
◆ press forcefully into the edge to apply pressure. Make each thrust distinct, with the intent to dislodge the obstruction.
◆ repeat thrusts until the obstruction is relieved

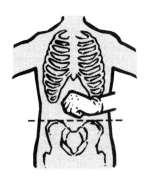

Abdominal thrusts

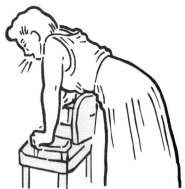

8

You are alone, eating your dinner. You suddenly find yourself choking on a piece of meat. From the following actions, check ☑ the procedures that could help you to cough up the piece of food.

- ☐ A. Drink a glass of water to wash down the food.
- ☑ B. Give yourself repeated, strong abdominal thrusts with your fist.
- ☑ C. Dial 911 immediately for medical help, if you can.
- ☑ D. Bend over the edge of your dining table and push sharply against your abdomen.
- ☐ E. Push your back several times against the wall.

9

Chest thrusts

When you are in the **late stages of pregnancy** or if you are **very obese,** abdominal thrusts cannot be applied effectively.

◆ Try to call for medical help or to attract attention

The following procedure creates a pressure similar to a chest thrust performed by a first aider:

◆ make a fist and place it thumb side down in the middle of your chest
◆ with your head turned to the side, fall against a wall hard enough to produce a chest thrust
◆ make each thrust distinct, with the intent to clear the obstruction
◆ repeat this procedure until the obstruction is relieved

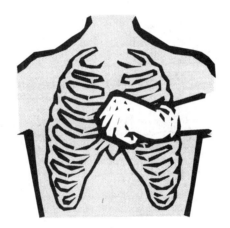

Chest thrusts

10

When you give first aid for choking, which of the following persons would require chest thrusts?

Check ☑ your choices.

☐ A. An average sized woman who is unconscious.
☑ B. A young man who is extremely overweight.
☑ C. A young woman in her last month of pregnancy.
☐ D. A very tall and muscular athlete.

B C

First aid for choking—review

· ·

11

The following questions are based on the videos, your practical exercises and this activity book exercise.

A choking person clutches her throat, is red in the face and is coughing forcefully and loudly.

From the first aid procedures shown below, check ☑ the appropriate action you should take.

☐ A. Landmark for abdominal thrusts.

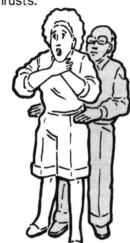

☑ B. Stand by and encourage coughing.

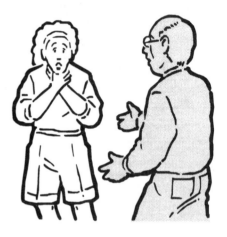

☐ C. Give up to five chest thrusts.

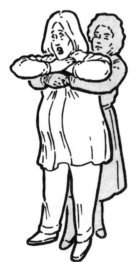

☐ D. Give up to five abdominal thrusts.

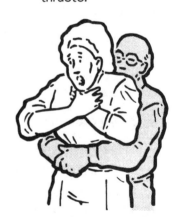

12

A choking person is conscious and has great difficulty breathing. Her lips are bluish and she is unable to answer your question, "Are you choking?"

From the first aid procedures shown below, check ☑ the one action you should take immediately.

☐ A. Use a hooked finger sweep in the casualty's mouth to remove the obstruction.

☐ B. Send for medical help immediately.

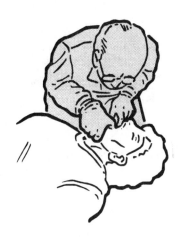

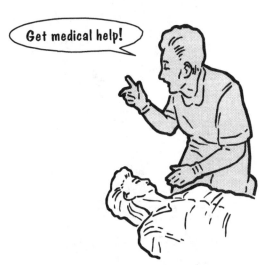

Get medical help!

☐ C. Encourage the casualty to cough up the obstruction.

☑ D. Give abdominal thrusts until the obstruction is relieved or the person becomes unconscious.

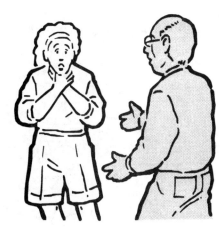

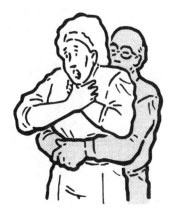

13

A conscious choking casualty becomes unconscious. Number the first aid actions for this casualty **in the order you should do them**. Place the appropriate number in the boxes provided.

5 A. Try to ventilate, reposition the head and try again.

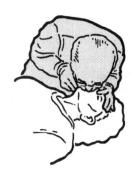

B. Ease her to the floor and call or go for medical help.

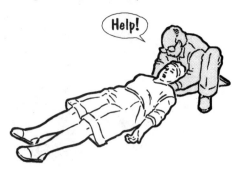

6 C. Landmark and give abdominal thrusts.

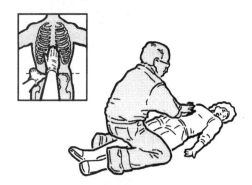

4 D. Open the airway.

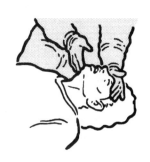

2 E. Open the mouth using the tongue-jaw lift.

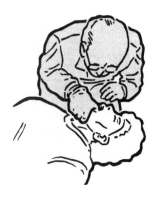

3 F. Finger-sweep the mouth.

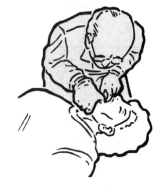

Ongoing casualty care until hand over

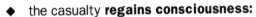

14

When a choking person's airway has been cleared and ...

- the casualty **remains conscious:**
  - ❖ monitor breathing and circulation frequently
  - ❖ stay with the casualty until breathing is well established and skin colour has returned to normal
  - ❖ urge the casualty to see a medical doctor

- the casualty **regains consciousness:**
  - ❖ monitor breathing and circulation frequently
  - ❖ give first aid for shock
  - ❖ stay with the casualty until medical help takes over
  - ❖ urge the casualty to see a medical doctor

- the casualty **remains unconscious:**
  - ❖ monitor breathing and circulation frequently and assist breathing if necessary
  - ❖ place the casualty into the recovery position
  - ❖ give first aid for shock
  - ❖ stay with the casualty until medical help takes over

Note: Choking manoeuvres can cause internal damage.

C A U T I O N

Breathing problems, and other signs of choking may be caused by swelling in the airway due to an allergic reaction to food or a bee sting, an infection or injury. Do not waste time trying to relieve this obstruction. Get medical help immediately.

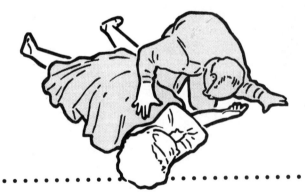

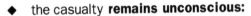

15

Check ☑ the correct completions to the following statement. When an airway obstruction has been removed by abdominal or chest thrusts, and normal breathing has been restored, the casualty should:

- ☐ A. Require no medical help.
- ☑ B. Be observed closely to ensure complete recovery.
- ☑ C. Be placed into the recovery position if not fully conscious.
- ☐ D. Be seen by a doctor to check for possible injuries.

Objectives

• •

Following the videos and upon completion of your practical skills and this activity book exercise, in an emergency situation you will be able to:

◆ take measures to prevent choking

◆ recognize choking

◆ provide first aid for a choking adult

◆ provide ongoing casualty care until hand over for a casualty whose airway has been cleared

For further information on first aid for choking, please refer to:
First on the Scene, the St. John Ambulance first aid and CPR manual, chapter 3, available through your instructor or any major bookstore in your area.

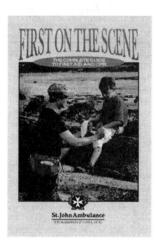

EXERCISE 5

SEVERE BLEEDING

8 min

Wounds

1

A **wound is any break in** the continuity of **the soft tissues** of the body.

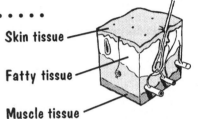

Skin tissue

Fatty tissue

Muscle tissue

A wound usually **results in bleeding.** Depending on the location of the wound, it may be either . . .

- ◆ **external bleeding:** blood escapes from the surface wound and can be seen, or
- ◆ **internal bleeding:** blood escapes from tissues inside the body and cannot be seen directly

Depending on the blood vessels that are damaged, bleeding can be either:

- ◆ **arterial bleeding:** blood is bright red and spurts with each heart beat from the damaged artery. Arterial bleeding is serious and often hard to control.
- ◆ **venous bleeding:** blood is dark red and flows steadily. It will stop more readily when being controlled.

Break in the continuity of the soft tissues

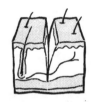

2

Mark each of the following statements as either true **(T)** or false **(F)**:

A. Loss of blood usually occurs when there is a break in the skin.

B. A deep cut on a finger is an example of a wound with internal bleeding.

C. When there are injuries inside the body, blood will leak into the surrounding areas.

D. Spurting blood is more difficult to stop than flowing blood.

E. Bleeding always looks the same, no matter where it comes from.

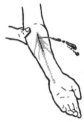

Arterial bleeding

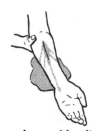

Venous bleeding

A.T B.F C.T D.T E.F

Signs and symptoms of bleeding

3

The sign of **external** bleeding is the **appearance of blood. Blood** is **not** immediately **visible** with **internal** bleeding.

General signs and symptoms of bleeding may vary widely, depending on the amount of blood loss. **Severe blood loss** will result in the following signs and symptoms:

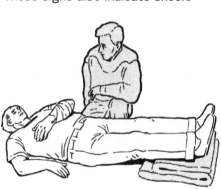

Wound with external bleeding

- ◆ pale, cold and clammy skin
- ◆ rapid pulse, gradually becoming weaker
- ◆ faintness and dizziness
- ◆ thirst and nausea
- ◆ restlessness and apprehension
- ◆ shallow breathing, yawning, sighing and gasping for air (known as air hunger)

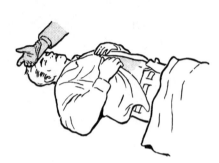

These signs also indicate shock.

4

Of the following, check ☑ the signs and symptoms that may appear when a casualty is bleeding severely from a deep cut into the thigh.

The casualty...

☐ A. feels light-headed and asks for a drink of water.

☐ B. has a hot flushed face and appears restless.

☐ C. is panting for breath and his skin is cool and moist to the touch.

☐ D. complains that he is about to vomit.

☐ E. has blood-soaked trousers and pooling of blood under his leg.

☐ F. has a strong, slow pulse.

A C D E

5

Internal bleeding may not be easy to recognize.

A casualty can bleed to death without any blood being seen.

Mechanisms of injury:

You should **suspect internal bleeding** when the following **mechanisms of injury** are apparent:

◆ the casualty has received a severe blow or a penetrating injury to the chest, neck, abdomen or groin

◆ there are major limb fractures or a hip or pelvic fracture

Suspect internal bleeding also with **certain medical conditions**, e.g. ulcers, hemophilia (bleeders).

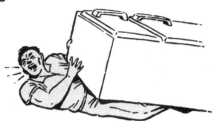

Crush injury

Characteristics of internal bleeding

Internal bleeding may **remain hidden**, or you may recognize it by one or more of the following **characteristic signs**:

Blood may be . . .

◆ discharged from the ear canal, the nose, or it may appear as a bloodshot or black eye

◆ red and frothy when coughed up

◆ seen in vomitus either as bright red, or brown like coffee grains

◆ appearing in the stools either as black and tarry, or in its normal red colour

◆ seen in the urine as a red or smoky brown colour

If bleeding is severe, **signs of shock** will be present.

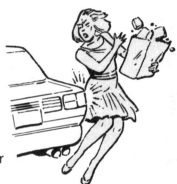

Fractured pelvis

6

Check ☑ the correct completions of the following statement:

You should suspect internal bleeding when the casualty:

☐ A. Has been punched hard in the stomach.

☐ B. Shows no signs of external bleeding, but has a cold, clammy skin, a rapid, weak pulse and is gasping for air.

☐ C. Had a finger partially cut off when slicing a loaf of bread.

☐ D. Coughs up bright red blood mixed with air bubbles.

☐ E. Shows reddish discolouration in the waste products from his body.

☐ F. Has obvious bleeding from a gaping wound on the leg.

Fractured upper leg
(femur)

A   B   D   E

First aid principles for severe external bleeding

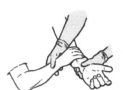

Direct pressure

7

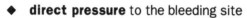

Severe bleeding is an immediate threat to life.
You must act quickly!
If bleeding remains uncontrolled, shock and death may result

Control severe bleeding by:

◆ **direct pressure** to the bleeding site

❖ Apply continuous pressure with your hand over a pad of dressings, or with the casualty's bare hand. You may have to bring the edges of the wound together before applying pressure if the wound is large and gaping

❖ Continue pressure by securing dressings with a firm bandage

❖ If dressings become blood soaked, do not remove them. Apply additional dressings and secure with fresh bandages

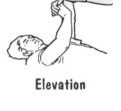

Elevation

◆ **elevation**

❖ If injuries permit, raise an injured limb above the level of the heart. This will help reduce blood flow to the wound

❖ Elevate an injured limb as much as the injury and the casualty's comfort will permit

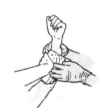

◆ **rest**

❖ Place the casualty at rest. The preferred position is lying with lower legs raised about 30 cm (12 inches) if injuries permit

Steady and **support** the injured part and give ongoing casualty care while awaiting medical help.

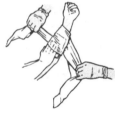

8

Your co-worker has cut his forearm on a sharp knife and blood is flowing freely from the wound.

Of the following actions, check ☑ the correct procedures you should take to control the bleeding.

☑ A. Tell the casualty to press firmly on the wound, raise his arm and lay him down, then go for the first aid kit.

☑ B. Place several layers of dressings on the wound and maintain pressure.

☐ C. Replace all wet dressings with dry ones.

☐ D. Lower the casualty's arm below heart level after you have applied the bandage.

☑ E. Provide support for the injured arm and continue to monitor the casualty's condition.

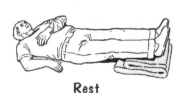

Rest

A B E

Impaired circulation

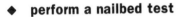

9

Some injuries and first aid procedures may result in reduced blood flow to the limbs:

◆ **injuries at, or close to, a joint** may pinch an artery

◆ **a bandage** that is too tight

◆ **injury to a major blood vessel**

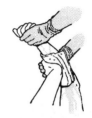

Checking temperature before bandaging

To check for impaired circulation below the injury:

◆ **compare** the **temperature** and **colour** of the injured limb below the injury (fingers or toes) to the uninjured limb before and after bandaging

  ❖ any drop in temperature in the limb is probably caused by a reduced blood flow

◆ **perform a nailbed test**

  ❖ press on a fingernail or toenail until it turns white

  ❖ release pressure; note how long it takes for the normal colour to return

  ❖ if it returns quickly, blood flow is good

  ❖ if it remains white or regains colour slowly, blood flow is impaired

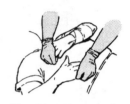

Checking temperature after bandaging

To improve impaired circulation caused by too tight bandages, you should immediately:

◆ **loosen the bandages**; if bleeding starts again, re-tie the bandages

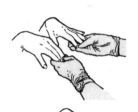

If circulation is still impaired:

◆ **obtain medical help** immediately

Continue checking circulation until hand over to medical help.

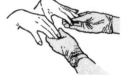

Nailbed test

10

You have bandaged a wound on a casualty's arm to maintain control of bleeding. When you recheck for circulation below the point of injury, you note that the hand is colder to the touch than on the uninjured arm and the tips of the fingers stay white when they are compressed.

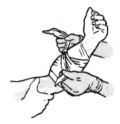

Untying bandage

Check ☑ what you should do for this casualty:

☐ A. Call medical help before doing anything else.

☑ B. Ease the tightness of the bandage and check for good circulation.

☐ C. Rub the fingers to get them as warm as the fingers of the other hand.

☑ D. Tighten the bandages again, if blood shows through the dressings.

☑ E. Call medical help right away if easing up the bandages does not help circulation.

B D E

Care of amputated tissue

11

In many cases amputated parts can be surgically reattached. Proper care of the amputated tissue, therefore, is very important.

For a completely amputated part, you should:

◆ wrap it in a clean, moist dressing, if possible; otherwise a clean and dry dressing
◆ place it in a clean, watertight plastic bag and seal it
◆ place it into another bag with a cold pack or crushed ice to keep it cool
◆ label the bag with the casualty's name, date and the time it was wrapped
◆ take or send the part to medical help with the casualty

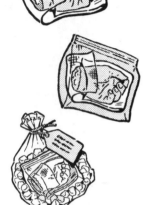

For a partially amputated part, you should:

◆ keep it as near as possible to its normal position
◆ cover it with a moist dressing if possible; otherwise a dry dressing. Apply direct pressure on the wound to stop bleeding
◆ secure the dressings in place with a bandage
◆ obtain medical help as soon as possible

Care of a completely amputated part

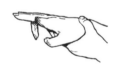 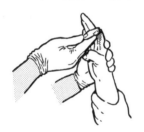 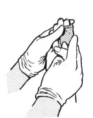 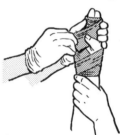 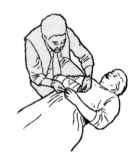

Care of a partially amputated part

12

Select and indicate ☑ the correct completions for the following statements.

A completely amputated part should be:

☑ A. Covered with a sterile, damp gauze, if available.
☐ B. Placed in a container with warm water to maintain body temperature.
☑ C. Sealed in a waterproof container and kept cool.
☑ D. Identified with the name of the first aider and the care given to the casualty.
☑ E. Sent to the hospital with the injured person.

A partially amputated part should be:

☑ F. Kept in its natural place with a dressing and bandage.
☐ G. Kept in place with adhesive tape.

A C E F

First aid for internal bleeding

13

The most important thing, you as a first aider, can do is to:

◆ **recognize** the history and mechanism of injury that might cause internal bleeding

◆ **recognize** shock

◆ give **first aid for shock** to lessen

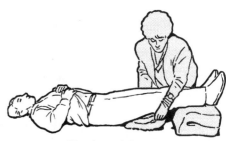

Shock position

its effects

◆ **obtain prompt medical help**

While waiting for medical help, make the casualty as comfortable as possible.

◆ Place the **conscious** casualty at rest on his back with feet and legs elevated to about 30 cm (12 inches), if injuries permit

◆ Place the **unconscious**, breathing casualty into the recovery position

◆ Reassure the casualty

◆ Preserve body heat

◆ Give nothing by mouth

◆ Reassess airway, breathing and circulation

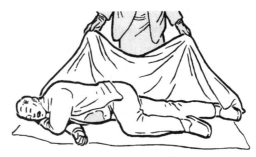

Recovery position

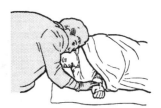

Recovery position covered

14

Which of the following would you do for a conscious casualty with suspected internal bleeding?

Check off ☑ your choices:

☐ A. Tell the casualty that he is bleeding badly inside his body.

☑ B. Obtain medical help quickly.

☑ C. Comfort the casualty with gentle encouragement.

☑ D. Place a blanket under and over the casualty.

☐ E. Allow the casualty to take sips of water.

☑ F. If the condition allows, raise the casualty's lower legs on a folded coat.

B   C   D   F

Objectives

· ·

Following the videos and upon completion of your practical skills and this activity book exercise, in an emergency situation, you will be able to:

◆ use dressings and bandages in first aid procedures

◆ recognize major wounds

◆ recognize severe external and internal bleeding

◆ provide first aid for wounds with severe external bleeding

◆ provide first aid for amputations and care for amputated tissue

◆ recognize inadequate circulation to the extremities and provide the appropriate first aid

◆ provide first aid for internal bleeding

For further information on first aid for severe bleeding, please refer to:
First on the Scene, the St. John Ambulance first aid and CPR manual, chapter 6, available through your instructor or any major bookstore in your area.

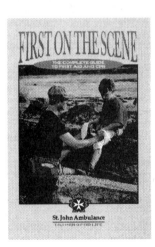

CARDIOVASCULAR EMERGENCIES

AND ONE RESCUER CPR—ADULT

The heart

1

The **heart** acts as a pump. It continuously circulates blood to the lungs and all parts of the body. To do this work, it needs a steady supply of blood rich in oxygen and nutrients.

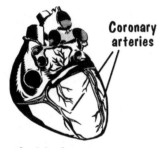

Coronary
arteries

Healthy heart

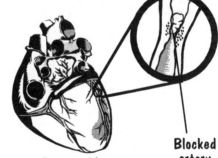

Blocked
artery

Damaged heart

Two **coronary arteries** supply this blood to the heart muscle. If the coronary arteries or their branches become narrowed or blocked, a part of the heart will not receive the oxygen it needs. This will cause a cardiovascular emergency.

2

Mark each of the following statements as either true (**T**) or false (**F**).

A. When the body is at rest, the heart does not require oxygen.

B. The heart sends blood to all parts of the body.

C. Special blood vessels provide oxygenated blood to the heart tissue.

D. A heart problem results when part of the heart muscle does not receive enough blood supply.

A.F B.T C.T D.T

8 - 1

Risk factors

. . . .

3

A **risk factor** is a behaviour or trait that increases the chance of someone developing cardiovascular disease. Some risk factors can be controlled, while others cannot.

Cardiovascular risk factors	
Can be controlled	**Cannot be controlled**
Cigarette smoking	A person's
Elevated blood cholesterol	– Age
Elevated blood pressure	– Gender
Diabetes	– Family history
Obesity	
Lack of exercise	
Excessive stress	

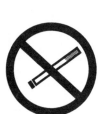

The risk of developing a cardiovascular disease can be reduced considerably by adopting a healthy lifestyle.

. . . .

4

Check ☑ the healthy lifestyle habits that can help control the risk of cardiovascular disease.

☑ A. Ensure a non-smoking environment for yourself and your family.
☑ B. Start an exercise program after consultation with your doctor.
☐ C. Eat food high in fat and calories.
☑ D. Have blood pressure checks by a health professional on a regular basis.
☑ E. Maintain a recommended body weight.
☑ F. Take time to relax and rest.
☐ G. Smoke a pipe instead of cigarettes.

A B D E F

Instructor-led exercise 8A

5

CARDIOVASCULAR DISEASE

High blood pressure (Hypertension)

1. _blood presure_ is the pressure of blood pushing against the inside walls of the blood vessels.

2. A person is said to have high blood pressure when his blood pressure is _constantly_ above normal.

3. Two effects of high blood pressure are:

    a) The walls of the blood vessels become _thick and less elastic_

    b) The heart becomes _enlarged_ .

4. The casualty with high blood pressure **always / almost never** shows signs and symptoms. *(Circle your choice.)*

Narrowing of Arteries (Atherosclerosis)

5. Narrowing of arteries is caused by a build up of ~~fat~~ _fatty deposits_ on the inside lining.

Narrowed artery

6. The process of fat being deposited in the arteries begins: *(Circle your choice.)*

    a) when angina begins   (b) in childhood)   c) in middle age.

7. In the coronary arteries the build up of fatty deposits results in _coronary artery disease_

Angina

8. Angina is a short-lived pain usually felt in the: *(Circle the correct answers.)*

    (a) chest)   b) neck)   c) shoulders)   d) jaw)   e) hips   f) arms)

9. Angina occurs when the heart does not get enough _oxygen_ to meet its needs.

10. The most common reason the heart does not get enough oxygen is that the arteries have become _a narrow_ .

Instructor-led exercise 8A (cont'd)

5

Heart attack

Blocked artery

11. A heart attack is most often caused by a _blood clot_ blocking a coronary artery that is already narrowed. The blood clot blocks the flow of blood to the _heart_.

12. Part of the heart muscle dies because it does not get the _oxygen_ it needs.

13. A heart attack often feels similar to _indigestion_.

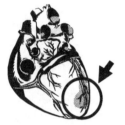

Damaged heart

Cardiac arrest

14. Cardiac arrest means that the heart has stopped _pumping blood_

15. Cardiac arrest is also called _sudden death_.

16. Common causes of cardiac arrest are:

a) _heart attack_   d) _poison_

b) _stroke_   e) _drowning_

c) _electricity_   f) _____

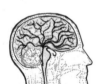

Healthy brain

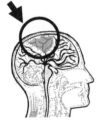

Damaged brain

Stroke

17. A stroke is a condition in which part of the brain tissue dies because of a shortage of _oxygen_.

18. A stroke can be caused by:

a) a _block_ in the circulation of blood to the brain; **or**

b) a ruptured blood vessel in the _brain_.

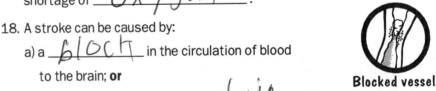

Blocked vessel

19. A transient ischemic attack (TIA), is a condition similar to a stroke. It is often called a "mini stroke". A TIA is of short duration and leaves no permanent damage. A TIA is a warning sign that a _stroke_ may follow.

Advise anyone who has a TIA to seek medical help.

Ruptured vessel

Answers: Addendum C

Angina/heart attack

6

Angina results from a temporary shortage of oxygen to the heart muscle. The signs and symptoms of angina are similar to a heart attack, except that they are often brought on by physical effort or stress and should be relieved by medication and rest. There is no heart damage in angina as there is in a heart attack.

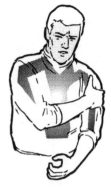

Pain in arm

Signs and symptoms of a heart attack

The casualty may **deny** that he is having a heart attack but you may recognize some or all of the following:

You may see:

◆ shortness of breath
◆ paleness, sweating, and other signs of shock
◆ vomiting
◆ unconsciousness

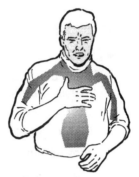

Shortness of breath

The casualty may complain of:

◆ crushing chest pain which may or may not be severe
◆ pain spreading to neck, jaw, shoulders and/or arms
◆ shortness of breath
◆ fear, feeling of doom
◆ feeling of indigestion
◆ nausea

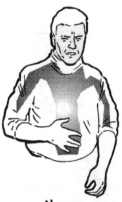

Nausea

If some or all of these signs and symptoms are present, a cardiac arrest may follow. Most heart attack deaths occur within the first two hours of the onset of signs and symptoms.

7

Which of the following signs and symptoms might help you to recognize angina or a heart attack? Check ☑ your answers from the listing below.

☐ A. A tingling sensation in the hands and feet.
☑ B. Breathing difficulty.
☑ C. Discomfort in the heart region.
☑ D. The casualty's insistence that it is just a stomach upset.
☐ E. A flushed face.
☑ F. White, moist skin.
☑ G. The casualty is frightened.

| B | C | D | F | G |

First aid for angina/heart attack

8

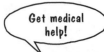

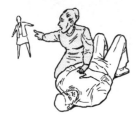

The first aid for angina and heart attack is the same.

Your aims for all cardiovascular emergencies are to:

◆ get medical help quickly

◆ reduce the workload of the heart

◆ prevent the casualty's condition from worsening

When you suspect that a person is having a heart attack or angina:

◆ get medical help **immediately**

◆ place the person at rest in the position of most comfort, usually **semisitting,** to ease the work of the heart and help breathing

◆ loosen tight clothing at the neck, chest and waist

◆ reassure the casualty

◆ assist the casualty to take prescribed medication, if requested

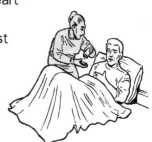

Assess breathing. If breathing fails, begin AR immediately.
Assess the pulse. If the pulse stops, begin CPR.

Helping the casualty to take medication

Only assist a casualty with medication if he is fully conscious and specifically requests your help.

Always check the five "rights" before assisting with medications:

◆ *right medication*

◆ *right person*

◆ *right amount*

◆ *right time*

◆ *right method*

9

A middle aged man collapses after running for a bus. He is pale and sweating, is clutching his chest, but is fully conscious. You suspect a heart attack. Which choice of action should you take?

Check ☑ your choices.

Choice 1

☐ A. Help him into his house.

☑ B. Prop up his head and shoulders with your coat.

☑ C. If he asks you, help him take his prescribed medicine.

☐ D. Tell him there is nothing to worry about.

☑ E. Provide AR and CPR if required.

Choice 2

☑ A. Send someone to call for an ambulance.

☐ B. Raise his legs with your coat.

☐ C. Give him plenty of water to drink.

☑ D. Speak to him gently and tell him help is on the way.

☐ E. Leave him as dead if breathing or the heart stops.

A.2 B.1 C.1 D.2 E.1

Cardiac arrest

10

Signs of a cardiac arrest

You will note:

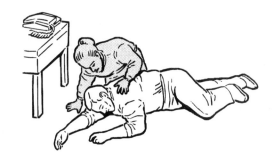

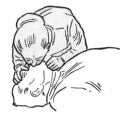

◆ unresponsiveness
◆ no breathing
◆ bluish colour
◆ no pulse

First aid for a suspected cardiac arrest

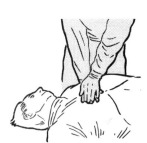

◆ Perform ESM
◆ Check ABC — airway, breathing and circulation (pulse)
◆ If there is no breathing and no pulse, **start cardiopulmonary resuscitation (CPR) immediately**

CPR is a combination of two life-support techniques, **artificial respiration** and **artificial circulation.**

The chain of survival

CPR is important, but it is only one of the five steps in the **chain of survival**. Each link is as important as the others. You, the first trained person on the scene, are the crucial first three links in the chain of survival:

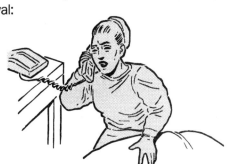

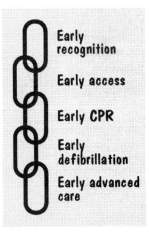

◆ **early recognition** of a cardiovascular emergency
◆ **early access** to emergency medical services (EMS); this means calling for help quickly
◆ **early CPR**
◆ **early defibrillation** given by emergency personnel
◆ **early advanced care** given by medical personnel

Early recognition
Early access
Early CPR
Early defibrillation
Early advanced care

11

From the options below, choose ☑ the condition which requires that you give CPR:

☐ A. The casualty is unresponsive but is breathing.
☑ B. The casualty is not breathing and has no pulse.
☐ C. The casualty is not breathing but has a pulse.
☐ D. The casualty is choking and has difficulty breathing.

Signs and symptoms of stroke

. . . .

12

The signs and symptoms of stroke differ depending on what part of the brain was damaged. You may note some or all of the following:

You may see:

◆ decrease in the casualty's level of consciousness
◆ paralysis of facial muscles
◆ difficulty in speaking and swallowing, e.g. slurred speech, drooling
◆ unsteadiness or a sudden fall
◆ loss of coordination
◆ loss of bladder and bowel control
◆ unequal size of pupils

Unequal size of pupils

The casualty may complain of:

◆ numbness or weakness of arms or legs, especially on one side
◆ severe headache

Paralysis of facial muscles (drooping of face)

. . . .

13

Check ☑ the signs and symptoms which could indicate that a stroke has occurred.

☑ A. The casualty wants to talk to you but cannot seem to get the words out.
☑ B. The casualty cannot move his left arm or leg.
☐ C. The casualty appears to be overactive and vomits.
☑ D. The casualty cannot control his need to urinate or move his bowels.
☐ E. When you check the pupils, they are the same size.
☑ F. You notice that the muscles on one side of the face are drooping.

A B D F

First aid for stroke

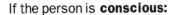

14

When you suspect that a person has had a stroke, you should **obtain medical help immediately.** Hospital treatment within one hour of the onset of symptoms will greatly increase the casualty's chances for recovery.

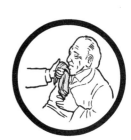

While waiting for medical help, you should:

◆ maintain adequate breathing and circulation

◆ protect him from injury

◆ reassure the casualty

◆ make him as comfortable as possible

◆ loosen tight clothing

If the person is **conscious:**

◆ place him at rest and support him in a **semisitting** position, unless the casualty has a weakness to one side of the body which prevents a semisitting position

◆ moisten his lips and tongue with a wet cloth, if he complains of thirst

If the person is **unconscious:**

◆ place him into the **recovery position** on the paralysed or weakened side to ease breathing

◆ give him nothing by mouth

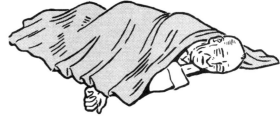
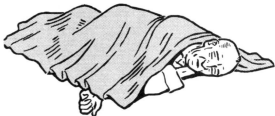

If breathing stops, begin AR immediately. If the heart stops, give CPR.

15

A middle-aged man suddenly becomes paralysed on his left side. He is conscious and has difficulty speaking. You suspect he has had a stroke.

Check ☑ the correct first aid actions you should take:

☑ A. Instruct someone to call for an ambulance.

☐ B. Tell him to speak clearly.

☑ C. Unbutton his shirt at the neck and loosen his belt.

☐ D. Give him a glass of water to drink.

☑ E. Position him on his left side to help his breathing.

☑ F. Take care to avoid further damage to his body.

A C E F

Cardiovascular emergencies—review

· ·

16

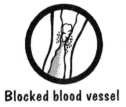

Blocked blood vessel

1. Depending on its location in the body, a blood vessel that is narrowed but not completely blocked, is most likely to cause which of the following cardiovascular emergencies?
   Check ☑ your answers.

   ☑ A. TIA (transient ischemic attack—little stroke)

   ☐ B. Stroke

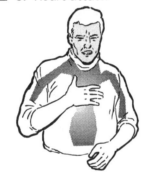

   ☐ C. Heart attack

   ☑ D. Angina

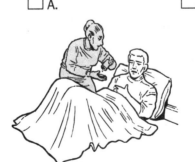

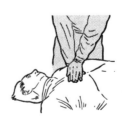

2. You have found a casualty who is not breathing and has no pulse. Which of the following illustrations shows part of the correct first aid procedures?
   Check ☑ your answer.

   ☐ A.   ☐ B.   ☐ C.

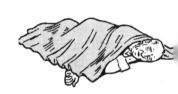

1.A 1.D 2.B

Cardiovascular emergencies—review
Instructor-led exercise 8B

17

What is happening	Signs & symptoms	First aid
Angina/Heart attack A1. The heart muscle is not getting enough blood through the coronary arteries to _____ _____ .	A3. Pain in the _____ . A4. Pain may _____ . A5. Any of the following: _dein_ , fear, paleness, nausea, _vamithy_ , indigestion, shortness of breath, unconsciousness, cardiac arrest.	A6. Perform a _Scene Survy_ A7. Perform a _primary. Sa_ A8. ____Go____ for medical help. A9. Place the casualty at rest in a comfortable position. Loosen tight clothing. A10. If requested, help the _Cov'nis'hay_ casualty to take prescribed medication. A11. Give ongoing casualty care until _Medhoal aid_ .
Heart attack A2. Part of the heart muscle is not getting enough blood through the coronary arteries to keep the _heart_ _tissue alive_.		
Cardiac arrest B1. The heart has _Stoppd_ and is not _pumpn_ any blood.	B2. Unconsciousness. B3. There is no _breathing_ . B4. There is no _pulse_ .	B5. Begin with a _Soan survy_ B6. Assess _Rroia on_ . B7. _Send_ for medical help. B8. Continue with a primary survey and start _CPR_ .
Stroke C1. A part of the _brain_ is not getting enough blood to function properly. With a stroke, brain tissue _dies_ . **TIA** C2. A part of the brain is not getting enough blood to function properly. With TIA, brain tissue _is OK_ .	C3. _Changes_ in level of consciousness. C4. _pupls_ of unequal size. C5. Hard to _speah_ and/or swallow. C6. Numb or _paralyzed_ arm or leg. C7. Mental confusion. C8. Convulsions. C9. The signs and symptoms of a _TIA_ are not long lasting.	C10. Perform a _Sean_ . C11. Perform a _primary_ C12. _Send_ for medical help. C13. Place the casualty at rest in a _Canforto'_ position. _Loosen_ tight clothing. C14. Give _novthy_ by mouth. C15. ____'____ the casualty during movement or convulsions. C16. If unconscious, place in _____ position, _____ side down. C17. Give ongoing casualty care until _____ .

Answers: Addendum C

Objectives

Following the videos and upon completion of your practical skills and this activity book exercise, in an emergency situation you will be able to:

◆ apply the knowledge of cardiovascular disease

◆ apply the knowledge of risk factors of cardiovascular disease

◆ apply the knowledge of preventive health measures

◆ apply the principles of first aid for cardiovascular emergencies

◆ recognize angina/heart attack and provide first aid

◆ recognize a cardiac arrest

◆ perform one-rescuer cardiopulmonary resuscitation (CPR) on an adult casualty

◆ recognize a stroke/TIA and provide first aid

For further information on cardiovascular emergencies and CPR, please refer to: *First on the Scene*, the St. John Ambulance first aid and CPR manual, chapters 5 and 11, available through your instructor or any major bookstore in your area.

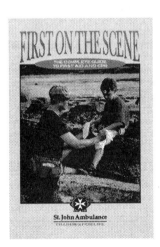

SECONDARY SURVEY

10 min

. . . .

1

Once you have given first aid for life-threatening conditions, you may need to do a secondary survey.

A secondary survey should be done when:

◆   medical help is delayed

◆   the casualty tells you about more than one area of pain

◆   you must transport the casualty to a hospital

The secondary survey is a step by step gathering of information which will help you to get a complete picture of the condition of the casualty.

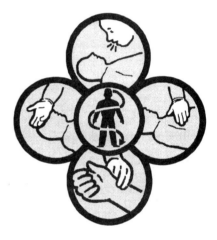

The secondary survey consists of four steps that you should do in the following order:

1.   obtain the history of the casualty

2.   assess and record vital signs

3.   perform a head-to-toe examination

4.   give first aid for injuries and illnesses found

. . . .

2

Mark each of the following statements relating to the secondary survey as either true **(T)** or false **(F)**:

☐ A. You do a secondary survey to discover any immediate danger to the casualty's life.

☐ B. Before you transport a casualty, you should check each part of his body carefully for signs of injuries.

☐ C. The steps of the secondary survey can be done in any sequence that is convenient.

☐ D. With the secondary survey you can find out details about the person's injuries and illnesses.

A.F B.T C.F D.T

3

History of the casualty

By taking the history of a casualty, you are trying to find out everything that is important about the casualty's condition.

A simple way to ensure that you take a complete history of the casualty, is to remember the word **SAMPLE,** where each letter stands for a part of the history:

S = symptoms

A = allergies

M = medications

P = past and present medical history

L = last meal

E = events leading to the incident

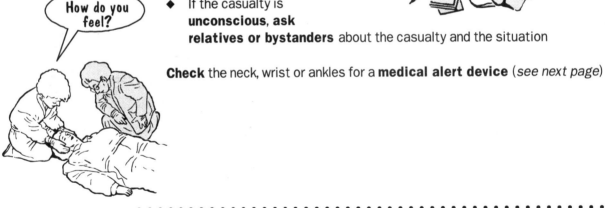

◆ **Ask the conscious casualty** how she feels now. Be guided by the casualty's complaints

Where do you hurt?

◆ If the casualty is **unconscious, ask relatives or bystanders** about the casualty and the situation

How do you feel?

Check the neck, wrist or ankles for a **medical alert device** (*see next page*)

4

If you want to find out about the history of the casualty, which of the following actions should you do?

Check ☑ the correct answers.

☐ A. Ask the conscious casualty where she feels pain at the moment.

☐ B. Question witnesses about what happened to the unresponsive casualty.

☐ C. Find out about the casualty's past history to help you give appropriate first aid.

☐ D. Ask bystanders what first aid to give.

Medical alert information

5

A **medical alert** device, e.g. a **bracelet, necklace, anklet or pocket card** contains valuable information about the medical history of a casualty. Sometimes this information is kept in a specially marked container on the top shelf of the **person's refrigerator.** Look on the refrigerator door for directions.

When examining an **unconscious** casualty **look for medical alert information.** It may help you in your assessment and in giving appropriate first aid. Some medical alert devices give a phone number where more information about the casualty can be obtained.

A medical alert device may **warn you** that a person wearing it –

◆ has a **medical condition** needing special treatment
or
◆ is **allergic** to certain substances, e.g. medications, foods, insect bites, plants

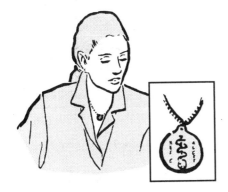

Medical alert necklace

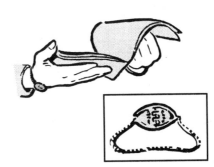

Medical alert bracelet

6

Mark each of the following statements as either true **(T)** or false **(F)**:

☐ A. Important facts that may affect the condition of a casualty may be revealed on a medical alert device.

☐ B. Medical-alert jewellery may be worn by a person whose arm swells and who has difficulty breathing after a bee sting.

☐ C. Medical alert information will tell you the age of the casualty.

☐ D. You should also search for medical alert information on every conscious casualty.

A.T B.T C.F D.F

7

Vital signs

The **vital signs** are important indicators of a casualty's condition. The four vital signs you will learn about are:

1. level of consciousness
2. breathing
3. pulse
4. skin condition

You should note and record the vital signs as a basis for further assessments.

Levels of consciousness (LOC)		
When a person is **conscious**	When a person is **semi-conscious**	When a person is **unconscious**

	When a person is **conscious**	When a person is **semi-conscious**	When a person is **unconscious**
Eye opening response	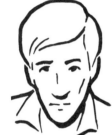 eyes open spontaneously	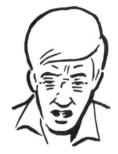 eyes open to speech or pain	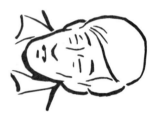 eyes don't open
Verbal response	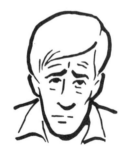 he is oriented and alert	he is confused, doesn't make sense	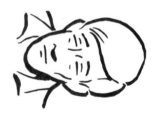 he is not aware of his surroundings
Motor response	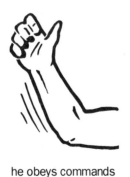 he obeys commands	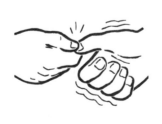 he reacts to pain	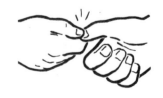 he doesn't react to pain

Any serious injury or illness can affect consciousness.

Levels of consciousness (cont'd)

Refer to chart with LOC on page 10 – 4

How to assess the level of consciousness
(Modified Glasgow Coma Scale)

You assess a person's level of consciousness by rating three of his responses:

1. **Eye opening response**	2. **Best verbal response**	3. **Best motor response**
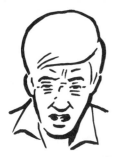	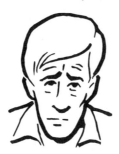	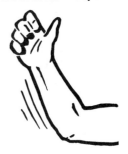
"Open your eyes"	*"What time is it?"*	*"Move your fingers"*

Any changes in the level of consciousness should be noted and recorded.

8

Match each casualty's description with a level of consciousness by writing the appropriate number into the squares provided.

Casualty

☐ A. A woman is lying on the street. She opens her eyes only when you talk to her, but is unable to tell you her name and where she lives.

☐ B. A child has fallen off his bicycle and is lying on the ground. As you approach, he starts to cry and reaches for his bicycle.

☐ C. After calling out to a man found lying on the floor and tapping his shoulders, he neither opens his eyes, nor answers.

Levels of consciousness

1. Conscious
2. Semi-conscious
3. Unconscious

A.2 B.1 C.3

9

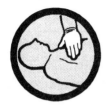

How to assess breathing

If the casualty **is conscious:**

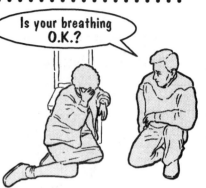

Is your breathing O.K.?

◆ **look** at the casualty's chest/abdomen and **ask**: "Is your breathing O.K.?"

◆ **listen** to how well the casualty answers and **note** the quality (rate, rhythm and depth) of breathing

If the casualty has difficulty responding, cannot respond, or **is unconscious:**

◆ **place** a hand on the chest of the casualty and

◆ **check the rate, rhythm and depth of breathing**

Normal, effective breathing is quiet and effortless with an even steady rhythm. Check for:

Is your breathing O.K.?

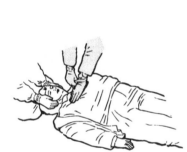

◆ **rate** – is the number of breaths per minute within the normal range?

◆ **rhythm** – are the pauses between breaths of even length?

◆ **depth** – is the breathing shallow, too deep or gasping and noisy?

The following table gives breathing rates for all ages. If a casualty's breathing is too slow or too fast, assist breathing with artificial respiration; see page 3 – 7 in this activity book.

Breathing rate — breaths per minute			
age group	range of normal rates	too slow	too fast
adult (over 8 yrs.)	10 to 20	below 10	above 30
child (1 to 8 yrs.)	20 to 30	below 15	above 40
infant (under 1 yr.)	30 to 50	below 25	above 60

10

From the examples below, check ☑ the signs that could help you determine if a casualty needs help with breathing.

☐ A. The casualty says that her breathing is fine.

☐ B. Breathing becomes laboured and noisy.

☐ C. The pauses between breaths change from very short to very long.

☐ D. Breathing is smooth and regular.

B C

11

How to assess the pulse

The pulse is the pressure wave with each beat of the heart that is felt at different parts of the body. By taking the pulse you check that the heart is beating and blood is circulating throughout the body.

When assessing the pulse, note the:

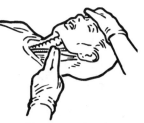

The carotid pulse

◆ **rate** – how many times does the heart beat in a minute?

◆ **rhythm** – are the pauses regular between the pulse beats?

◆ **strength** – are the pulse beats strong or weak?

Normal pulse rates, by age	
age	rates (heartbeats per min.)
adult (8 and over)	50 to 100
child (1 to 8)	80 to 100
infant (under 1 yr.)	100 to 140

The pulse of a healthy adult at rest varies from 50 to 100 beats , **averaging about 72 beats per** minute, is strong, and has a regular rhythm.

Never use your thumb

to take a pulse—it has

a pulse of its own and

you may feel it instead

of the casualty's pulse.

How to determine your own pulse rate carotid/radial:	
1. Feel your pulse	
2. Count the number of beats for 30 seconds	
3. Multiply by 2	x 2
4. The result is **your pulse rate**	

Pulse rates for an adult at rest (beats per minute)

slow	normal range	fast
40 50 60	70 72 80 90	100 110 120

↑
average

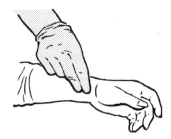

The radial pulse

Does your pulse rate fall within the **normal** range for an adult?

12

Mark the following statements regarding the pulse as either true **(T)** or false **(F)**:

☐ A. The presence of a pulse indicates that the person is breathing normally.

☐ B. The radial pulse can be checked on either wrist.

☐ C. The pulse can be taken on more than one location of the body.

☐ D. A pulse count of 68 beats per minute in a resting adult casualty is within a normal range.

A.F B.T C.T D.T

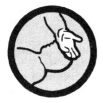

13

Skin condition and temperature

The condition and temperature of the skin change when there is shock. Checking skin condition and temperature will help you to find out if the casualty is in shock.

How to assess skin condition

◆ check the skin for colour –
   ❖ is it pale, reddish or bluish?
◆ check for presence of sweat –
   ❖ is the skin clammy or dry?

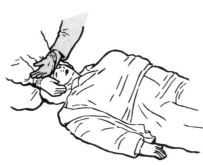
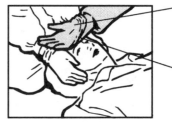

place the back of your hand on the forehead, neck or cheek

pull back your glove if necessary to feel change of temperature

How to assess skin temperature

◆ use the back of your hand which is more sensitive to feel –
   ❖ is the skin warm, hot or cool?
   ❖ is the skin dry or wet?

Reassess the vital signs every few minutes or when you think the casualty's condition has changed. Write down your findings and the time of each observation.

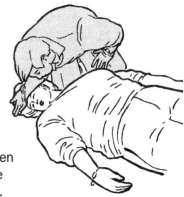

14

From the choices below, check ☑ the correct answer to the following question.

When assessing skin condition and temperature, which one of the following groups of signs would indicate shock (inadequate circulation to body tissues)?

☐ A. Red, hot and dry skin.
☐ B. Pale, cold and clammy skin.
☐ C. Red, hot and sweaty skin.
☐ D. Bluish, cold and dry skin.

Head-to-toe examination—review

· ·

15

The following question is based on the video and your practical exercise.

In the secondary survey you should examine a casualty from head-to-toe for less obvious injuries and illnesses. What sequence in the **top-down approach** would you follow to ensure a **thorough, systematic** examination of the casualty?

Place the illustrations **in the order** you have learned to do the head-to-toe examination by writing the appropriate number into the squares provided:

☐ A. Check the neck.

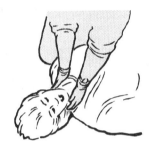

☐ B. Check the head.

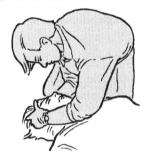

☐ C. Check the shoulders, arms and hands.

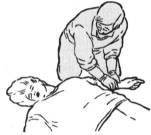

☐ D. Check the chest and under.

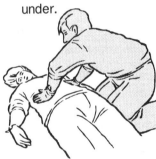

☐ E. Check both collar-bones.

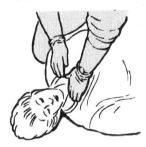

☐ F. Check the pelvis and buttocks.

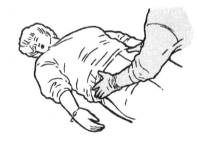

☐ G. Check the abdomen and under.

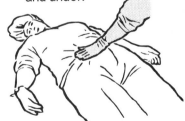

☐ H. Check the legs, ankles and feet.

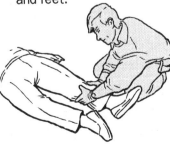

Give first aid for injuries and illnesses found.

A.2 B.1 C.4 D.5 E.3 F.7 G.6 H.8

Objectives

· ·

Following the video and upon completion of your practical skills and this activity book exercise, in an emergency situation, you will be able to:

◆ perform the four steps of a secondary survey:

 ◆ obtain the history of the casualty

 ◆ assess and record vital signs

 ◆ perform a head-to-toe examination

 ◆ give first aid for non life-threatening conditions

For further information on the secondary survey, please refer to:
First on the Scene, the St. John Ambulance first aid and CPR manual, chapter 2, available through your instructor or any major bookstore in your area.

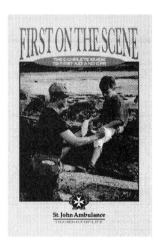

BONE & JOINT INJURIES

6 min

—UPPER LIMBS; MUSCLE STRAINS

Fractures

· ·

1

A basic knowledge of the structure of the upper limbs will help you to give first aid for injuries to these parts of the body.

A **fracture** is any break or crack in a bone.

A fracture may be **closed** or **open**

◆ **Closed fracture** – a fracture where **the skin is not broken**

◆ **Open fracture** – a fracture where **the skin is broken** and **bone ends may protrude**

The cause/mechanism of injury for upper limb fractures may be:

◆ **direct force**, e.g. a hard blow or kick

◆ **indirect force**, e.g. the bone breaks at some distance from the point of impact

◆ **twisting,** e.g. abnormal turning (rotation) of shoulder or wrist joint

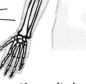

Upper arm (humerus)

Forearm (radius and ulna)

Upper limb

· ·

2

Mark each of the following statements as either true **(T)** or false **(F)**.

☐ A. There is one long bone between the shoulder and the elbow.

☐ B. There are two separate, long bones between the elbow and the wrist.

☐ C. A cracked bone over which the skin is swollen is considered an open fracture.

☐ D. A fracture over which a bleeding wound is seen is a closed fracture.

☐ E. A broken collarbone that results from a fall on the outstretched arm is caused by indirect force.

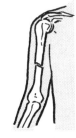

Closed fracture

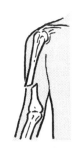

Open fracture

A.T B.T C.F D.F E.T

Joint injuries

. . . .

3

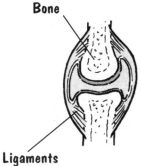

Bone

Ligaments

Joint with supporting tissue (ligaments)

A **joint** is formed where two or more bones come together. Joints allow for body movement. The bones of a joint are held in place by supporting tissue called **ligaments**.

The major joints of the upper limb are at the:

◆ shoulder

◆ elbow

◆ wrist

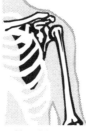 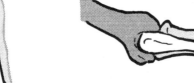 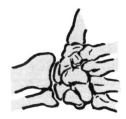

Shoulder joint   **Elbow joint**   **Wrist joint**

Joint injuries happen when the bones and surrounding tissues are forced to move beyond their normal range.

Two common joint injuries are **sprains** and **dislocations**:

◆ **sprain** – a complete or partial tearing or stretching of the ligaments around a joint

◆ **dislocation** – a displacement of one or more bone ends at a joint so that their surfaces are no longer in proper contact

. . . .

4

Mark each of the following statements as either true **(T)** or false **(F)**.

☐ A. A joint is where two or more bones meet.

☐ B. Tissues surrounding the bones of a joint prevent its movement.

☐ C. A sprain occurs when the supporting tissues around a joint are over-stretched or damaged.

☐ D. A dislocation occurs when the bones at a joint are pushed out of their position.

A.T B.F C.T D.T

General signs and symptoms

5

Some or all of the following signs and symptoms occur in most bone and joint injuries –

You may see:

♦ swelling and discolouration
♦ deformity and irregularity
♦ protruding bone ends
♦ inability to use the limb
♦ guarding and tensing of muscles around the injured area
♦ grating noise that can be heard as the bone ends rub together
♦ signs of shock, increasing with the severity of the injury

The casualty may complain of:

♦ pain made worse by movement
♦ tenderness on touching

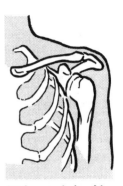

Dislocated shoulder

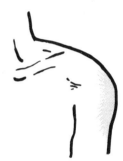

Deformity and swelling of the shoulder

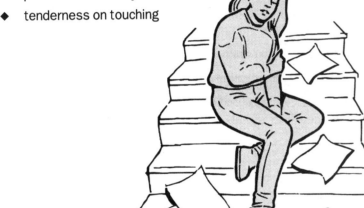

Shoulder dislocation

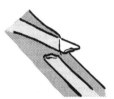

Open fracture of the humerus

6

Which of the following could indicate a bone or joint injury of the upper limb?

Check ☑ the correct answers.

☐ A. A cut on the upper arm is bleeding profusely.
☐ B. The end of a bone is sticking through the skin of the forearm.
☐ C. A casualty is pale and sweating. His skin feels cold and his shoulder is in an unnatural position.
☐ D. A casualty cannot bend his elbow and screams when you touch it.
☐ E. A hockey player has fallen and has a painful, swollen wrist.

B C D E

Principles of first aid

7

The **aims of first aid** for bone and joint injuries are:

◆ to prevent further damage and reduce pain

The first aid principles to be followed are:

For any closed fracture, sprain or dislocation, keep the casualty as comfortable as possible with:

◆ *R - Rest*

◆ *I - Ice*

◆ *C - Compression/ bandaging*

◆ *E - Elevation*

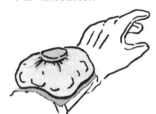

◆ perform a scene survey
◆ do a primary survey and give first aid for life-threatening injuries
◆ treat the injury at the incident site, if possible
◆ control bleeding from open wounds, if present
◆ if medical help is close by, **steady and support the injured part** in the position of greatest comfort
◆ apply a cold compress, a wrapped, cold pack or ice bag on any closed fracture or injury to reduce pain and control swelling (15 minutes on – 15 minutes off)
◆ apply gentle pressure/compression with a bandage to reduce swelling
◆ elevate the injured part, if possible
◆ monitor the casualty closely for any change in his condition
◆ reassure the casualty
◆ do not give anything to eat or drink
◆ give ongoing casualty care until hand over

Note: ◆ All fractures, dislocations and sprains should be immobilized before the casualty is moved, unless the casualty is in immediate danger

8

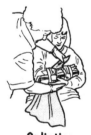

Splinting

Match each situation with the first aid procedure you should perform. Place the appropriate number into the boxes provided:

First aid procedures	Situations
☐ A. Splinting	1. Medical help is readily available.
☐ B. Steady and support	2. A wound over the fracture site is bleeding.
☐ C. Expose and bandage	3. You have to transport the casualty to the hospital.

Expose and bandage

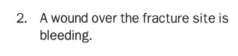

Muscle strains

. . . .

9

A **strain** is an injury that occurs when a muscle is stretched beyond its normal limits.

The cause/mechanism of injury for a strain may be:

◆ sudden pulling or twisting of a muscle
◆ poor body mechanics during lifting
◆ failure to condition muscles before physical activity
◆ repetitive, long-term overuse

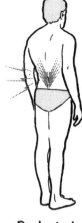

Back strain

A strain can be recognized by some or all of the following –

You may see:

◆ swelling of muscle
◆ discolouration

The casualty may complain of:

◆ sudden sharp pain
◆ severe cramps
◆ stiffness

Signs and symptoms may not appear until later.

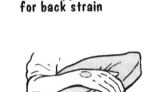

**Position of comfort
and cold application
for back strain**

To give first aid, you should:

◆ place the casualty in the position of greatest comfort
◆ apply cold (15 minutes on – 15 minutes off) to help relax muscle spasm, reduce pain and prevent further tissue swelling
◆ refer to medical help

Repetitive strain injury (RSI) is a term that refers to a number of injuries, including back injuries, joint injuries, tennis elbow and bursitis. It is caused by long-term overuse of some joints, muscles and support tissue.

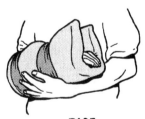

Position of comfort

To give first aid:

◆ keep the casualty as comfortable as possible with
◆ rest, ice, compression and elevation—think RICE
◆ refer to medical help

Prevention: Work breaks, exercises, relaxation techniques, observing proper posture and use of personal protective equipment (wrist/back supports) are the keys to preventing repetitive strain injury.

. . . .

10

Mark each of the following statements as either true **(T)** or false **(F)**.

☐ A. A strain is damage to any of the body's joints.
☐ B. Back strain can be caused by improper carrying techniques.
☐ C. Use of an ice pack and rest is effective treatment for a back strain.
☐ D. A strained leg muscle may cause pain several hours later.

RICE

R — rest
I — ice
C — compression/
      bandaging
E — elevation

A.F B.T C.T D.T

Objectives

· ·

Following the videos and upon completion of your practical skills and this activity book exercise, in an emergency situation, you will be able to:

◆ recognize bone and joint injuries

◆ provide first aid for bone and joint injuries of the upper limbs

◆ recognize muscle strain and provide first aid

◆ recognize repetitive strain injury and provide first aid

For further information on bone and joint injuries of the upper limbs, and muscle strains, please refer to: *First on the Scene*, the St. John Ambulance first aid and CPR manual, chapter 7, available through your instructor or any major bookstore in your area.

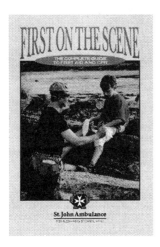

HEAD/SPINAL AND PELVIC INJURIES

Introduction to head/spinal and pelvic injuries

1

A basic knowledge of the structure of **the head, spine** and **pelvis** and **how they relate to each other**, will help you to understand how injury to one part may affect the other part. It will help you to give the appropriate first aid.

Injuries to the head, spine and pelvis are always serious because of the **danger of injury to the nervous system.**

The nervous system is made up of the:

◆ brain
◆ spinal cord
◆ nerves

These delicate tissues are protected by the:

◆ skull
◆ spine

All body functions are controlled by the nervous system. The pelvis is a basin-shaped bony structure connected to the base of the spine.

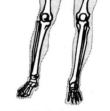

Skull

Spine

Pelvis

Nervous system

Full skeleton

2

Mark each of the following statements as either true **(T)** or false **(F)**.

☐ A. A blow to the head may cause brain damage.
☐ B. The bony parts of the head and backbone protect the soft parts beneath.
☐ C. The spinal cord and the brain are independent from each other.
☐ D. An injury to the pelvis may involve an injury to the lower part of the spine.

A.T   B.T   C.F   D.T

When to suspect head/spinal injuries

· ·

3

The **history/mechanism of injury** is the **first indication** that can lead you to suspect head/spinal injuries.

Head/spinal injuries should be suspected when a casualty:

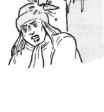

- ◆ has fallen from a height or down the stairs
- ◆ has been in a car collision
- ◆ has received a blow to the head, spine or pelvis
- ◆ has blood or straw-coloured fluid coming from the nose or ears
- ◆ is found unconscious and the history is not known

The **injuries** that are commonly **associated** with a **head injury** are **neck and spinal injuries.**

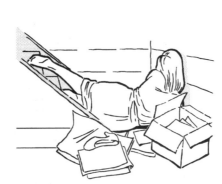
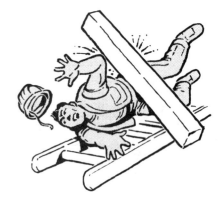

Mechanisms of injury

· ·

4

In which of the following circumstances should you suspect that the casualty has suffered head/spinal injuries?

Check ☑ the correct answers.

- ☐ A. A boy hits his head when he dives into a shallow pool.
- ☐ B. A young person is found unconscious in bed with an empty bottle of sleeping pills on the floor.
- ☐ C. A heavy wooden crate falls from a hoist and hits a worker on the back.
- ☐ D. During a collision, the knees of a person strike the dashboard with great force.

How to recognize head/spinal injuries

. . . .

5

You can recognize head/spinal injuries by **signs and symptoms.**

You may see:

◆ changes in level of consciousness
◆ unequal size of pupils
◆ loss of movement of any part
◆ unusual lumps on the head or spine
◆ bruising of the head, especially around the eyes and behind the ears
◆ blood or straw-coloured liquid coming from the ears or nose
◆ vomiting

Unequal size of pupils

The casualty may complain of:

◆ severe pain or pressure in the head, neck or back
◆ tingling or loss of feeling or movement in the fingers or toes
◆ nausea
◆ headache

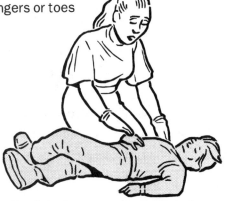

Checking for signs of spinal injuries

. . . .

6

When you are examining a casualty, which of the following signs and symptoms may indicate head/spinal injuries? Check ☑ the correct answers.

The casualty:

☐ A. Has a big bump on the bony area at the back of the head.
☐ B. Can feel when you squeeze his hand.
☐ C. Can make a fist and wiggle his toes when asked to do so.
☐ D. Tells you of prickling sensations in his hands and feet.
☐ E. Doesn't know what happened and wants to throw up.
☐ F. Has a yellowish fluid dripping from his nose and ears.

A D E F

Principles of first aid for head/spinal injuries

7

When a casualty has head/spinal injuries, **head or neck movement may lead to life-long disability or death.**

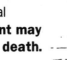

Don't move!

I know first aid, can I help you?

- ◆ Begin scene survey
- ◆ When the **mechanism of injury** suggests possible head/spinal injuries, tell the casualty **NOT TO MOVE**
- ◆ Offer to help and obtain consent from the conscious casualty
- ◆ **Send** for medical help **immediately**

Advanced medical attention within 1 hour can help avoid permanent damage following spinal injuries

- ◆ **Steady and support** the head and neck in the **position found**
- ◆ Assess responsiveness
- ◆ Check the airway and for breathing
- ◆ If you have a bystander, show him how to steady and support the casualty's head and neck
- ◆ If alone, **remind the casualty not to move**
- ◆ Continue to perform primary survey
- ◆ Give first aid for life-threatening conditions
- ◆ Give ongoing casualty care

Continue manual support of the casualty's head and neck in the position found until medical help takes over.

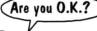

Are you O.K.?

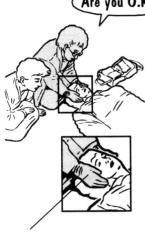

Firmly support the head and neck in the position found

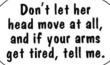

Don't let her head move at all, and if your arms get tired, tell me.

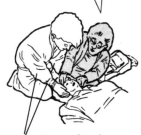

Keep elbows firmly supported on thighs or ground

8

Mark each of the following statements as either true (**T**) or false (**F**):

- ☐ A. A casualty may be hurt for life as a result of damage to the spinal cord and nerves.
- ☐ B. You should avoid any unnecessary moving of a casualty with suspected head/spinal injuries and obtain medical help promptly.
- ☐ C. The mechanism of injury is not important for the assessment and first aid for a head/spinal injury.
- ☐ D. You should caution a conscious person with suspected back injuries to remain as calm as possible.

A.T B.T C.F D.T

9

Maintain an open airway

Your **first aid priority** is maintaining an open airway and breathing.

If the casualty is not breathing:

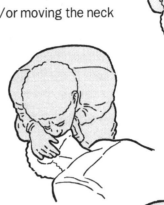

◆ **open** the airway, using the **jaw-thrust without head-tilt,**
this opens the airway without tilting the head and/or moving the neck

◆ give artificial respiration

◆ use your cheek to seal the casualty's nose if you do not have a mask to ventilate

◆ monitor breathing closely

If the casualty begins to **vomit:**

◆ **steady and support the head and neck**

◆ **turn** the casualty **as a unit** onto the side with as little movement of head and spine as possible

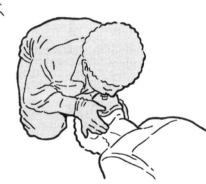

◆ quickly clear out the mouth

◆ reposition the casualty, **supporting her head and neck at all times**

◆ reassess breathing and pulse

◆ resume ventilations if required

◆ give ongoing casualty care until hand over

◆ **continue to support the casualty's head and neck** manually until medical help takes over

10

Check ☑ the correct completions for the following statements by writing the appropriate numbers into the squares provided.

When giving artificial respiration to a casualty with a suspected neck injury –

A. The head and neck should:

☐ 1. Be tilted backward.
☐ 2. Be tilted forward.
☐ 3. Not be tilted.

B. When the casualty starts vomiting:

☐ 1. Roll the casualty to the side keeping the head and neck in the same relative position with the body.
☐ 2. Turn only the head quickly to the side.
☐ 3. Leave the casualty on her back and try to clear the mouth.

A.3 B.1

Bleeding from a scalp wound

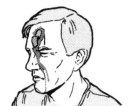

11

Bleeding from the scalp may be severe even if the wound is superficial. Any scalp wound, depending on the mechanism of injury, could indicate a serious head injury that may cause unconsciousness and breathing problems. If you suspect head/spinal injuries, tell the casualty not to move. If a bystander is available, ask him to steady and support the head and neck in the position found.

To control bleeding from a scalp wound (no head/spinal injury suspected):

- ◆ perform a scene survey
- ◆ determine the mechanism of injury
- ◆ wash your hands or put gloves on, if available
- ◆ perform a primary survey and give first aid for life-threatening conditions
- ◆ clean away loose dirt from the wound
- ◆ avoid direct pressure, probing or contaminating the wound
- ◆ apply a thick, sterile dressing large enough to extend well beyond the edges of the wound
- ◆ hold dressing in place with a triangular bandage
- ◆ get medical help promptly
- ◆ give ongoing casualty care until hand over

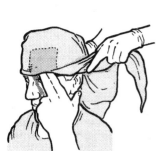

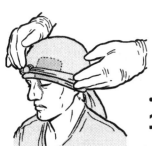

12

A conscious, breathing casualty is bleeding severely from a scalp wound. Before getting medical help for the casualty, what first aid should you do to control the bleeding?

Check ☑ the correct answers.

- ☐ A. Ask the casualty to maintain gentle pressure on the wound while you bandage.
- ☐ B. Cover the wound with a small adhesive dressing and secure it loosely in place.
- ☐ C. Apply large, soft dressings to the wound and secure them in place with a head bandage.
- ☐ D. Look for hidden dirt inside the wound and pick it out with your fingers.

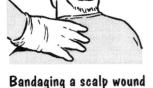

Bandaging a scalp wound

A C

Bump on the head

. . . .

13

A bump on the head is a very common injury, especially in children. It may be harmless. However, as any head injury, it should be taken seriously because of the possibility of injury to the brain.

To give first aid, for a bump on the head:

- be guided by the mechanism of injury
- if you suspect head/spinal injuries, tell the casualty not to move
- if you don't suspect head/spinal injuries, keep the casualty at rest
- put a cold compress or ice bag (15 minutes on – 15 minutes off) on the bruise to relieve pain and control swelling
- check the casualty often for:
  - ❖ changes in the level of consciousness (ask him questions, e.g. what his name is, where he lives)
  - ❖ a change in breathing, pulse and skin temperature
  - ❖ headache, nausea or vomiting
  - ❖ blood or straw-coloured fluid coming from the ears or nose
  - ❖ seizures
- if you see any of these signs or symptoms developing, even after many days, get medical help immediately

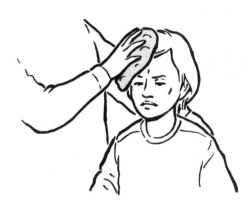

. . . .

14

Mark each of the following statements as either true **(T)** or false **(F)**.

- ☐ A. A person who has hit his head could have injured his brain.
- ☐ B. A person who is confused after a fall on the head should be observed carefully.
- ☐ C. You should apply heat to the bruised area.
- ☐ D. If the casualty's breathing becomes slow and laboured, you should get medical attention immediately.
- ☐ E. Any discharge from the ears could be a sign of a serious head injury.

A.T B.T C.F D.T E.T

Bleeding from the ear

● ●

15

Bleeding from the ear can have different causes. Bleeding, accompanied by a straw-coloured fluid, may indicate a fracture of the skull. To give the appropriate first aid, you have to **establish the mechanism of injury**.

If head / spinal injuries are not suspected:

◆ perform a scene survey
◆ perform a primary survey and give first aid for life-threatening conditions
◆ check for the cause of bleeding
◆ secure a dressing loosely over the ear
◆ place the conscious casualty semisitting, inclined toward the injured side
◆ place the unconscious casualty into the recovery position on the injured side
◆ obtain medical help
◆ give ongoing casualty care until hand over

Applying dressing

Positioning

If head / spinal injuries are suspected:

◆ perform a scene survey
◆ tell the casualty **not to move**. If a bystander is available, ask him to **steady and support the head and neck in the position found**
◆ do a primary survey and give first aid for life-threatening conditions
◆ make no attempt to stop the flow of blood or other fluids
◆ do not pack the ear with gauze
◆ place a dressing loosely over the ear
◆ check breathing frequently
◆ obtain medical help immediately
◆ give ongoing casualty care until medical help takes over

● ●

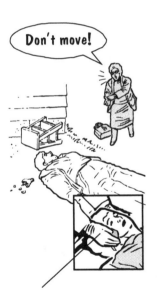

Don't move!

firmly support the
head and neck in the
position found and
apply dressing

16

From the following statements, check the correct choices for giving first aid when blood is oozing from a conscious casualty's ear.

When head / spinal injuries are suspected:

☐ A. Ask the casualty to stay completely still in the position found.
☐ B. Tape gauze dressings lightly over the ear.
☐ C. Support the casualty in a semisitting position.

When no head / spinal injuries are suspected:

☐ D. Tape gauze dressings lightly over the ear.
☐ E. Place the casualty into the recovery position.

A B D

Head/spinal injuries—review

. . . .

17

1. Which of the following illustration show a mechanism of injury that would indicate possible head/spinal injuries? Check ☑ your answers.

☐ A.

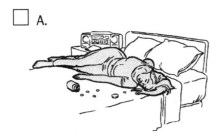

☐ B.

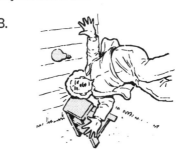

☐ C.

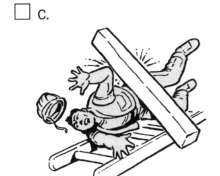

☐ D.

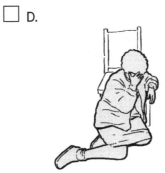

2. If you suspect head/spinal injuries, which of the following illustrations shows the right way to open the airway? Check ☑ your answer.

☐ A. Jaw-thrust without head-tilt

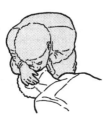

☐ B. Head-tilt chin-lift

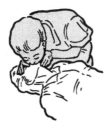

3. Which of the following illustrations shows the best positioning for a casualty with head/spinal injuries? Check ☑ your answer.

☐ A.

☐ B.

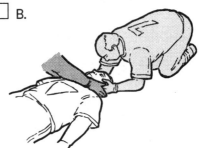

1.B 1.C 2.A 3.B

When to suspect a pelvic injury

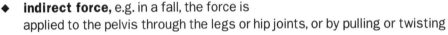

18

A **pelvic injury** is any break or crack in the bones of the pelvis.

When arriving at an emergency scene, look for the causes and the history of the incident. Try to find out what happened to the casualty's body and how much force was involved.

The mechanism of injury for a pelvic injury is usually:

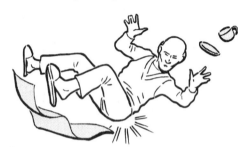

◆ **direct force,** e.g. a direct crush or heavy impact and may involve injury to the organs in the pelvic area, especially the bladder

◆ **indirect force,** e.g. in a fall, the force is applied to the pelvis through the legs or hip joints, or by pulling or twisting

In the elderly, even a simple fall may cause a fracture in the pelvic area.

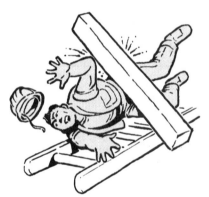
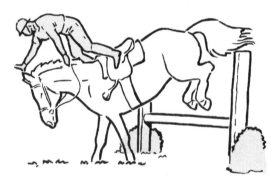

Mechanisms of injury

19

Mark each of the following statements as either true **(T)** or false **(F)**.

☐ A. To suffer a broken pelvis, a person must receive a blow right on the pelvic bones.

☐ B. A violent crushing of the knees against the dashboard in a car collision can result in a pelvic fracture.

☐ C. The pelvis is a strong, thick structure which is rarely injured in people over 60 years of age.

☐ D. A construction worker who has fallen from a ladder and landed on his feet may have injured his pelvis.

A.F B.T C.F D.T

Signs and symptoms of a pelvic injury

20

If the pelvis has been injured –

You may see:

◆ signs of shock (internal bleeding may be present)

◆ inability of the casualty to stand or walk

◆ inability to urinate or bloody urine

The casualty may complain of:

◆ sharp pain in the hips, groin and the small of the back

◆ increased pain when moving

◆ urge to urinate

An injury of the pelvis may result in damage to the **lower spine** or to the **bladder,** leading to serious infection.

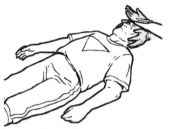

Check for shock

If you suspect a pelvic injury, do not squeeze the hips together.

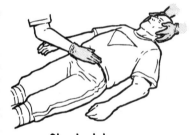

Check abdomen

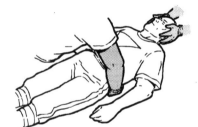

Check lower back

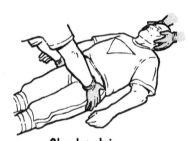

Check pelvis

21

Of the following statements, check ☑ the conditions of a casualty which may indicate a pelvic fracture.

☐ A. Strong discomfort around the pelvic area.

☐ B. The passing of pinkish urine.

☐ C. Pallor, sweating and a rapid pulse.

☐ D. Deformity of the feet.

☐ E. Moving around freely.

A   B   C

Principles of first aid for a pelvic injury

22

A **pelvic injury** is often **associated with a spinal injury** and should be treated with the same care as a spinal injury:

◆ begin scene survey
◆ when the mechanism of injury suggests a pelvic injury, tell the casualty **NOT TO MOVE**
◆ offer to help and obtain consent from the conscious casualty
◆ send for medical help immediately
◆ steady and support the casualty in the position found
◆ assess responsiveness
◆ check the airway and for breathing
◆ if there is a bystander, show him how to steady and support the casualty
◆ if alone, remind casualty not to move
◆ continue with the primary survey
◆ give first aid for any life-threatening condition
◆ **support both sides of the pelvis with padded objects to prevent movement**, e.g. rolled blankets
◆ give ongoing casualty care

Continue to support the casualty manually until medical help takes over.

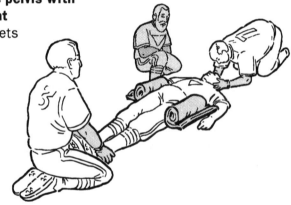

23

The mechanism of injury and the signs and symptoms indicate that the casualty is suffering from an injured pelvis. Medical help has been called and will arrive soon. What first aid should you give in the meantime?

Check ☑ the correct answers.

☐ A. Place the casualty in the recovery position.
☐ B. Tell the casualty to remain as still as possible.
☐ C. Place a rolled blanket on each side of the pelvis to keep the casualty from moving sideways and causing more pain.
☐ D. Reassure the casualty, maintain body heat and keep the casualty from moving until the ambulance arrives.

First aid for pelvic injuries—review

24

A baseball player was hit with a baseball bat in his lower back. He complains about sharp pain in the hips and in the small of the back. There are several bystanders ready to help.

Based on the history and mechanism of injury, number the correct first aid procedures for this casualty, **in the order you should perform them,** by placing the appropriate numbers into the squares provided.

☐ A. Take charge.

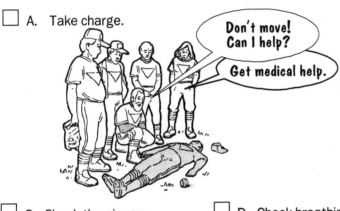

Don't move!
Can I help?

Get medical help.

☐ B. Support the pelvis.

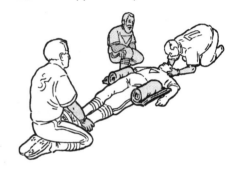

☐ C. Check the airway.

☐ D. Check breathing.

☐ E. Steady and support head and neck.

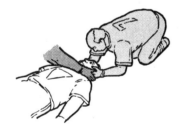

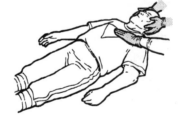

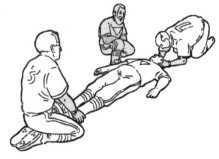

☐ F. Do a rapid body survey.

☐ G. Check for shock.

☐ H. Give ongoing casualty care.

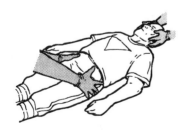

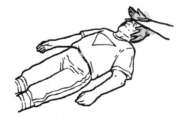

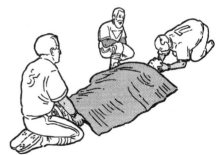

A.1 B.7 C.3 D.4 E.2 F.6 G.5 H.8

Objectives

• •

Upon completion of this activity book exercise, in an emergency situation, you will be able to:

◆ **recognize head/spinal injuries**

◆ **provide first aid for suspected head/spinal injuries**

◆ **control bleeding from the scalp and ear**

◆ **recognize a pelvic injury**

◆ **provide first aid for a suspected pelvic injury**

For further information on head/spinal and pelvic injuries, please refer to:
First on the Scene, **the St. John Ambulance first aid and CPR manual, chapter 7, available through your instructor or any major bookstore in your area.**

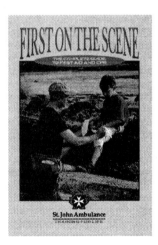

EYE INJURIES

Structure of the eye

1

The **eye** is the **very delicate** organ of sight. To give safe and appropriate care, you should know the **basic structure of the eye**.

Eyeball   – fluid-filled globe which is the main part of the eye

Cornea   – thin, transparent front of the eyeball that allows light to enter the eye

Eyelid   – movable layers of skin that provide a protective covering for the eye

Any injury to the eye is potentially serious and may result in **impaired vision** or **blindness.** Your quick response and the **correct first aid may help prevent permanent damage to the eye.**

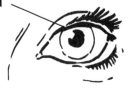

Front view of the eye

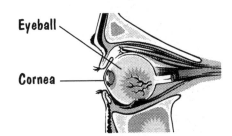

Cross section of the eye

2

Mark each of the following statements as either true **(T)** or false **(F)**.

☐ A. The eyeball is a hard, solid structure resistant to injury.

☐ B. Closing the eyelid protects the eye against entry of most foreign materials.

☐ C. The cornea is the delicate outer layer of the eye that can be seen from the front.

☐ D. An eye injury can cause complete or partial loss of sight.

☐ E. Loss of vision caused by an injury can often be avoided by prompt first aid.

A.F B.T C.T D.T E.T

Eye protection

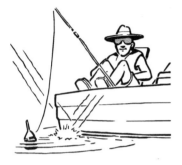

3

Eye protection helps to prevent eye injuries.

At home, at play or at work, you should adopt the following **safety practices**:

◆ wear safety glasses or a face shield when you work with tools or dangerous chemicals

◆ keep chemicals off high shelves and take care to avoid splashes

◆ wear eye protection when you play sports such as squash, racquetball or hockey

◆ wear dark glasses with UV 400 protection or a wide-brimmed hat in sunlight or when light reflects from snow or water

◆ avoid looking into bright lights such as an arc welding flash or an eclipse of the sun

4

Which of the following illustrations show practices that would help prevent eye injuries? Check ☑ the correct answers.

☐ A.

☐ B.

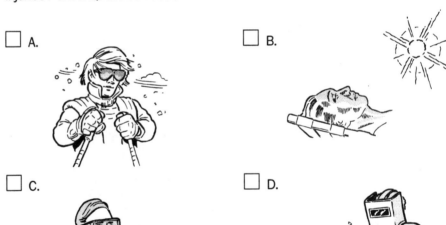

☐ C.

☐ D.

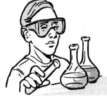

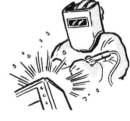

☐ E.

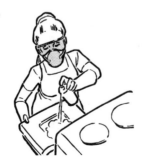

Particles in the eye

5

Particles, such as sand, grit or loose eyelashes, may enter the eye causing pain, redness or watering of the eye.

Never attempt to remove a particle from the eye when:

◆ it is on the cornea

◆ it is adhering to or embedded in the eyeball

◆ the eye is inflamed and painful

To locate and remove a **loose** particle, you may need **to examine the eye**. Follow these **general rules:**

◆ warn the person not to rub her eyes

◆ wash your hands and put gloves on

◆ stand beside the casualty and steady her head

◆ spread the eyelids apart with your thumb and index finger

◆ shine a light across the eye, not directly into it

◆ look for a shadow of the particle

If the particle on the eyeball, **is loose and not on the cornea**:

◆ try to remove it with the **moist corner** of a clean facial tissue or cloth

◆ if pain persists after removal, cover the eye and obtain medical help

Note: If the casualty is wearing contact lenses, let her remove the lens—then continue with first aid.

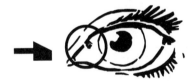

Particle on the eyeball

6

A small grain of sand has entered a person's eye. The tears have not washed it away. Which of the following techniques should you use to remove this grain from the eyeball? Check ☑ the correct answers.

☐ A. Give first aid for eye injuries with clean hands and in a good light.

☐ B. Seat the casualty with her back to a lamp to keep the light out of her eyes.

☐ C. Ensure that the object in the eye is floating freely.

☐ D. Hold the eyelids apart and use a damp end of a clean handkerchief to lift out a visible, loose grain.

A   C   D

7

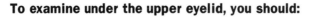

If tears do not wash away a small, loose object, and the particle is causing pain **under the upper lid:**

- ◆ ask the person to pull the upper lid down over the lower lid. The eyelashes on the lower lid may brush away the particle.

If your first examination does not locate the particle in the eye, you should examine under the eyelids.

To examine under the upper eyelid, you should:

- ◆ seat the casualty facing a good light
- ◆ wash your hands and put gloves on, if available
- ◆ stand beside the casualty
- ◆ steady the head and ask the casualty to look down
- ◆ place a cotton-tipped applicator stick at the base of the upper eyelid and gently press the lid backwards, but **don't press** on the eye
- ◆ grasp the upper eyelashes between the thumb and index finger
- ◆ draw the lid away from the eye, up and over the applicator stick and roll the applicator back

Pulling upper lid down

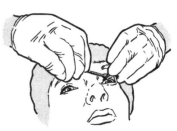

Upper lid drawn up

If the particle is visible:

- ◆ remove it with the moist corner of a clean facial tissue or cloth
- ◆ if pain persists after removal, cover the eye and obtain medical help

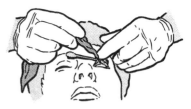

Remove a loose particle from under the upper eyelid

8

From the following statements, select the correct techniques for removing a loose particle from under the upper eyelid. Place a checkmark ☑ into the boxes provided.

- ☐ A. Tell the person to pull the top eyelid over the bottom one if the grain is under the top lid.
- ☐ B. Stand near the casualty's shoulder on the injured side.
- ☐ C. Instruct the casualty to roll the eyeball upward.
- ☐ D. Expose the underside of the upper eyelid by rolling the lid back.

If you can see the loose object:

- ☐ E. Try to lift it out with the moistened edge of a clean tissue.
- ☐ F. If discomfort persists, place a warm wet pad over the eye.

A B D E

9

To **look** for a loose particle from **under the lower eyelid,** you should:

◆ wash your hands and put gloves on

◆ seat the casualty facing a light

◆ gently draw the lower eyelid downwards and away from the eyeball while the casualty rolls the eyes upward

If the particle is visible:

◆ wipe it away with the moist corner of a facial tissue or a clean cloth

◆ if pain persists after removal, obtain medical help

If a particle does not become visible during your examination and the irritation persists, do not continue your attempts.

◆ Cover the **injured eye** with an eye pad or gauze and tape loosely in place

◆ Obtain medical help **immediately**

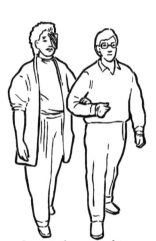

Remove loose particle from under lower lid

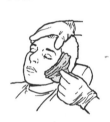 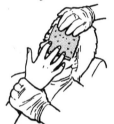 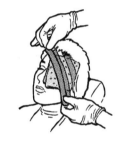

Covering the injured eye

Note: The reason for **covering the injured eye only** is to reduce psychological stress. If both eyes are injured, cover the eye that is most seriously injured. If both eyes must be covered due to serious injury in both eyes, e.g. intense light burn from arc welding, reassure the casualty often and explain what it is being done and why.

10

From the statements below, select the correct techniques for examining under the lower eyelid. Place a checkmark ☑ into the appropriate boxes.

☐ A. Tell the person to sit down.

☐ B. Seat the casualty with the back to a light.

☐ C. Pull the lower eyelid over the upper eyelid.

☐ D. Tell the person to roll the eyeball up.

If you are unsuccessful in finding the particle under the upper or lower eyelid, what should you do next?

☐ E. Repeat the examination until you find the object.

☐ F. Secure a soft dressing over the injured eye and take the person to the nearest medical facility.

Assist the casualty to walk

A D F

Objects adhering to or embedded in the eye

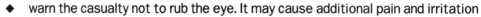

11

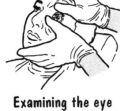

Examining the eye

When a **particle** (small object) or a **large object** is stuck to or is embedded in the eye or in the soft tissues near the eye, **do not attempt to remove it.**

You should:

◆ warn the casualty not to rub the eye. It may cause additional pain and irritation

◆ lay the casualty down and support the casualty's head to reduce movement (if available, use a bystander)

◆ wash hands and put on gloves, if available

Depending on the size of the object, use one of the following bandaging techniques.

First aid for a small embedded object or adhered particle:

◆ close the casualty's eyelids and cover the affected eye with a soft eye or gauze pad

◆ extend the covering over the forehead and cheek to avoid pressure on the eye

◆ secure lightly in place with a bandage or adhesive strips

◆ keep the casualty's head immobilized

◆ obtain medical help or transport lying down

◆ give ongoing casualty care until hand over

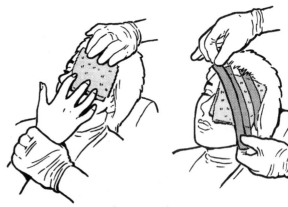

Covering the eye

Note: Do not try to remove a contact lens if there has been an injury to the eye other than a chemical burn.

12

Mark each of the following statements, dealing with first aid for an embedded particle in the eye, as either true **(T)** or false **(F)**.

☐ A. Ask the casualty not to touch the affected eye and to keep the head still.

☐ B. Use a cotton-tipped applicator to lift out a particle embedded in the eyeball.

☐ C. Place the casualty in a sitting position before you start bandaging.

☐ D. Secure a large, soft dressing loosely over the eye making sure that it does not press on the object.

☐ E. Cover both eyes to reduce the casualty's stress.

A.T B.F C.F D.T E.F

13

First aid for a large embedded object:

◆ lay the casualty down

◆ place dressings around the embedded object, using the "log-cabin technique" (building up dressings around the object) to prevent movement and tape in place

◆ ensure that there is no pressure on the embedded object

◆ immobilize the head to prevent movement

◆ transport the casualty on a stretcher to medical help

◆ give ongoing casualty care until hand over

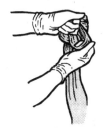

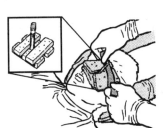

Log-cabin technique

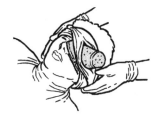

Cup and bandage

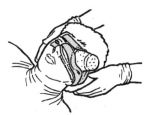

Taped cup

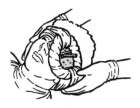

Ring pad bandage

Options for stabilizing an embedded object

How to prepare a ring pad bandage

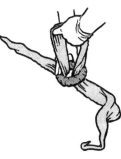

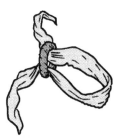

14

From the following statements, check ☑ the actions which describe the correct first aid for a large embedded object in the eye.

☐ A. Build up dressings around a large embedded object to keep it stabilized.

☐ B. Make sure that the casualty's head is kept still.

☐ C. Place a gauze square with a hole in the centre over the embedded object.

☐ D. Cover the injured eye only, to avoid more stress for the casualty.

☐ E. Help the casualty walk to the nearest medical facility.

A   B   D

Wounds to the eye

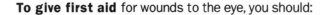

15

A **wound or bruise about the eye** is always serious because there may be underlying damage.

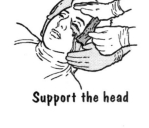

Support the head

A **bruise to the soft tissues** around the eye is usually the result of a blow from a blunt object. The bruise may not appear immediately, but there may be damage to the surrounding bones and internal structures. **A wound to the eyeball** from a sharp object is serious because of the possible damage to eyesight. **A wound to the eyelids** may cause **injury to the eyeball**. These wounds usually bleed profusely because of the rich blood supply.

To give first aid for wounds to the eye, you should:

- lay the casualty down, supporting the head, to prevent unnecessary movement
- wash your hands and put gloves on, if available
- close the eyelid and cover the injured eye lightly with a soft eye or gauze pad and tape in place
- apply a dressing to the area if there is bleeding. This will usually control it
- **never** apply pressure to the eyeball
- obtain medical help or transport on a stretcher with the head supported
- give ongoing casualty care until hand over

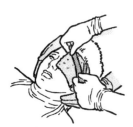

Cover the eye

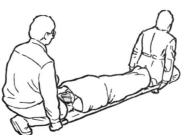

Tape gauze in place

Transport lying down

16

From the following statements, select the correct first aid for wounds near the eye. Place a checkmark ☑ into the appropriate boxes.

- ☐ A. Place the casualty at rest and prevent the head from moving.
- ☐ B. Heavy bleeding from the eye should be controlled with direct pressure.
- ☐ C. When bleeding from an eyelid has stopped, leave the dressing in place and bandage the injured eye.
- ☐ D. You should bandage a bruised eye tightly to stop the internal bleeding.
- ☐ E. When giving first aid for wounds to the eye, you should avoid pressing on the eyeball.

A C E

Extruded eyeball

. . . .

17

Severe injury may force the eyeball out of its socket.

Give first aid as follows:

◆ wash hands and put gloves on, if available

◆ **do not try to replace the eye into the socket**

◆ cover the extruded eyeball gently with a moist dressing and a cup and bandage

◆ obtain medical help. If not available,

❖ place the casualty face up on a stretcher with the head immobilized for transportation to medical help

❖ give ongoing casualty care until hand over

Serious injury could result if the casualty is not kept quiet and moved with great care.

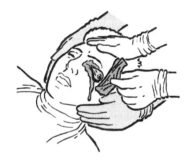 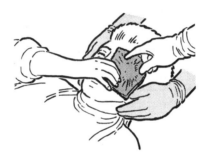

Moist gauze applied

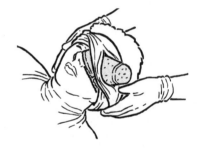

Cup and bandage

. . . .

18

A hockey player's eye was forced out of its socket when a puck hit his eye. Before immobilizing the casualty on a stretcher, which first aid procedures should you take?

Check ☑ your choices.

☐ A. Support the eyeball with a firmly applied dressing and bandage.

☐ B. Lay the casualty on a stretcher face up.

☐ C. Apply a damp dressing loosely over the extruded eyeball and cover it with a cup and bandage.

☐ D. Secure a damp gauze square also over the uninjured eye.

☐ E. Obtain medical care immediately.

B C E

Burns to the eye

• •

19

Eyes can be injured by **corrosive chemicals** (acids or alkalis). Chemical liquids or solids can cause **serious burns.** Casualties usually suffer intense pain.

The aim of first aid is to eliminate and dilute the chemical immediately. **You must act quickly!**

◆ Wash hands and put gloves on, if available

◆ Sit the casualty down with the head tilted back and turned slightly toward the injured side

If the chemical that entered the eye is a **dry powder**, you should first:

◆ brush the chemical away from the eye with a clean, dry cloth. Do **not** use your bare hands

◆ protect the uninjured eye

◆ gently force the casualty's eyelids apart

◆ flush the eye with tepid or cool water for **at least 15 minutes;** flush away from the uninjured eye

◆ cover the injured eye with dressings

◆ when both eyes are affected, cover only the more seriously injured eye, unless the casualty is more comfortable with both eyes covered

◆ get **immediate** medical help

Note: ◆ If the casualty wears contact lenses, ask her to remove them after flushing. If unable to do so, make sure medical help is notified.

◆ Proper eye irrigation equipment should be near at hand when there is a high risk of eye injury from chemicals.

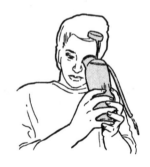

Commercial eyewash bottle

• •

20

Corrosive lime powder has blown into a person's eyes. Place the following first aid steps into the correct order of performance by placing the appropriate number in the boxes provided.

☐ A. Guide the person to an eye wash fountain and flush her eyes for approximately a quarter of an hour.

☐ B. Quickly remove any loose, dry powder from the face.

☐ C. Get the casualty to a medical facility immediately.

☐ D. Tape gauze squares over the eye which is more seriously hurt.

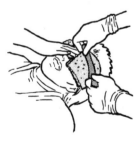

Intense light burns

. . . .

21

Burns to the eyes may be **caused by intense light** such as sunlight reflecting off snow, arc welder's flash or laser beams. Intense light burns **may not be painful at first** but may become very painful several hours after exposure.

When a casualty complains of burning in the eyes after exposure to bright, intense light, you should:

◆ wash hands and put gloves on, if available
◆ cover both eyes with thick, moist, cool dressings
◆ secure them in place (tape or narrow bandage)
◆ reassure the casualty as she is temporarily blinded
◆ obtain medical help
◆ give ongoing casualty care until hand over

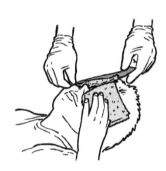

Cover eyes with moist gauze and tape in place

or

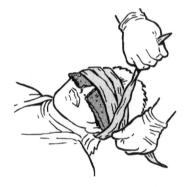

Secure moist gauze pads in place with narrow bandages

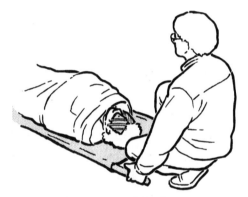

Transport with both eyes covered

. . . .

22

A welder suffers light burns to her eyes when she is not wearing her face shield. What first aid should you give?

Check ☑ the correct answer.

☐ A. Apply dry sterile dressings and take the casualty to medical aid.
☐ B. Place the casualty at rest in a cool darkened room until her pain lessens.
☐ C. Keep her eyes uncovered and allow the tears to cool them.
☐ D. Secure cool compresses to the eyes and transport the casualty to a medical facility.

Heat burns to the eyelids

· ·

23

When a casualty suffers burns to the face from fire, the eyes usually close as a natural reflex to protect the eyes. **Eyelids** may be burned and **need special care.**

First aid for burned eyelids:

◆ wash your hands or put gloves on, if available

◆ cover the eyelids with moist, cool dressings. The casualty will be temporarily blinded, so you must reassure her often and explain what you are doing. If the casualty doesn't want both eyes covered, even after an explanation and reassurance, cover only one eye

◆ secure in place

◆ call for medical help immediately

◆ give ongoing casualty care until hand over

Remember—when there is an injury to an eyelid, there may also be an injury to the eyeball.

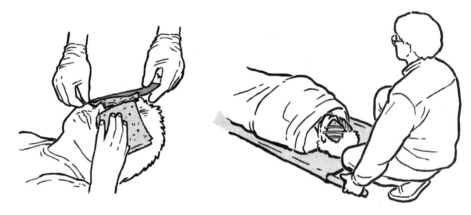

Cover both eyes with moist gauze

Transport lying down

· ·

24

Mark each of the following statements as either true **(T)** or false **(F)**.

☐ A. Burns to the eyelids are not considered serious and don't require medical treatment.

☐ B. Part of the first aid for burned eyelids is to apply several layers of dressings which have been soaked in cool water.

☐ C. Nature protects the eyeballs from heat by cooling them with tears.

☐ D. The application of cool, damp dressings to burned eyelids reduces the skin temperature and relieves pain.

A.F B.T C.F D.T

Eye injuries—review

· ·

25

1. A person complains of a dust particle under her upper eyelid. Which of the illustrations below show the correct first aid procedures?
   Check ☑ your answers.

☐ A.

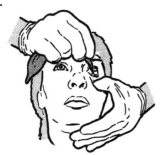

☐ B.

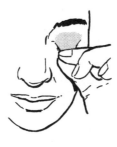

☐ C.

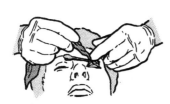

☐ D.

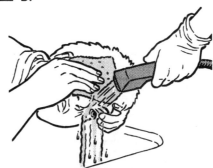

2. If you were unable to remove the particle, which of the following illustrations shows the correct eye covering you should use?
   Check ☑ your answers.

☐ A.

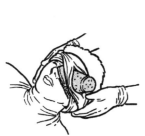

☐ B.

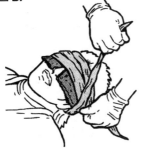

☐ C.

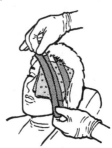

1.B 1.C 2.C

Objectives

• •

Following the video and upon completion of this activity book exercise, in an emergency situation, you will be able to:

◆ take measures to prevent eye injuries

◆ provide first aid for foreign objects in the eye

◆ provide first aid for wounds in and around the eye

◆ provide first aid for burns to the eye

For further information on first aid for eye injuries, please refer to:
First on the Scene, the St. John Ambulance first aid and CPR manual, chapter 6, available through your instructor or any major bookstore in your area.

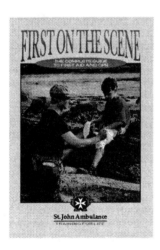

EXERCISE 19

BURNS

12 min

The skin

1

A basic knowledge of the skin and underlying tissues will help you to understand the serious damage **burns** can do and **to give appropriate first aid.**

Depending on the depth of the burn, the following tissues can be damaged:

◆ top layer of the skin (epidermis)
◆ second layer of the skin (dermis)
◆ fatty tissue
◆ muscle tissue

The skin **protects** the body against injury, extreme temperatures and infection.

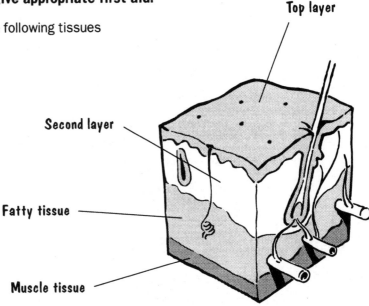

Top layer

Second layer

Fatty tissue

Muscle tissue

Skin and underlying tissues

2

Mark each statement below as true **(T)** or false **(F)**.

☐ A. Burns first destroy the outer part of the skin.
☐ B. The skin guards the body against outside damage.
☐ C. The skin is not affected by very hot temperatures.
☐ D. Burns break the skin and can cause serious problems.

A.T   B.T   C.F   D.T

Prevention of burns

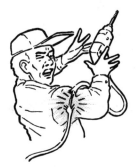

3

Burns are a leading cause of injury in the home, particularly among elderly people and young children. The diagrams below show you **dangerous situations** that may result in a burn.

Prevent burns by paying attention to the symbols shown on labels of hazardous products . . .

Danger corrosive   Danger flammable   Danger explosive   Danger radiation

and by adopting the following **safety measures:**

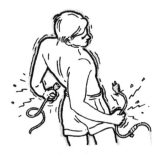

◆ use hand protection when you touch hot objects or work with corrosive chemicals

◆ keep electric equipment in good repair

◆ store flammable materials in a well-ventilated area

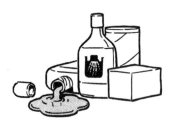

◆ clearly label corrosive and flammable chemicals or radioactive materials and store them in a safe place

◆ do not smoke in bed

◆ supervise children and elderly persons around hot stoves and when bathing

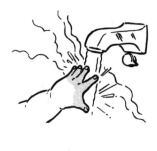

◆ install smoke alarms and fire extinguishers in your home and check them as suggested by the manufacturer

◆ develop and practise a fire escape plan

◆ wear protective clothing when exposed to radiation

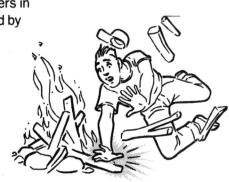

◆ protect yourself from sunburn by wearing a hat and sunscreen lotion

◆ wear sunglasses when outside in bright light

◆ be cautious around open fires

◆ wear non-flammable clothing

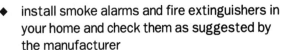

Types of burns

4

Burns cause damage to the skin and other underlying tissues.

The types of burns are grouped by their mechanism of injury (cause):

- ◆ **heat** – dry heat
  - – moist heat
  - – friction
- ◆ **corrosive chemicals**
- ◆ **electric current**
- ◆ **radiation** – sun rays
  - – radioactive materials

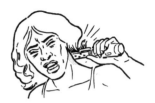

Dry heat

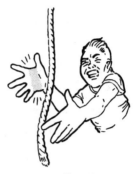

Friction

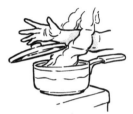

Moist heat

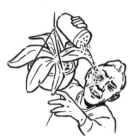

Corrosive chemicals

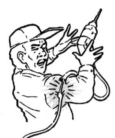

Electric current

5

In each of the following situations, a person is burned. Match each burn with one of the five causes by writing the appropriate number into the squares provided.

Situations	Causes
☐ A. A girl gets a sunburn while sleeping on the beach.	1. Dry heat
☐ B. A child in the bath is burned by hot water.	2. Moist heat
☐ C. A mechanic spills battery acid on his arm.	3. Corrosive chemicals
☐ D. A man receives burns when he uses a frayed electric cord.	4. Friction
☐ E. A woman is burned as a fire starts in the frying pan.	5. Electric current
☐ F. A boy's hands are burned when he loses his grip on a heavy rope.	6. Radiation

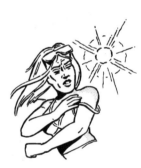

Sun rays

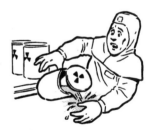

Radioactive materials

A.6 B.2 C.3 D.5 E.1 F.4

Signs and symptoms of burns

6

Signs and symptoms of burns depend on the depth of the burn. The **depth** of a burn is described as the degree of the burn.

First degree burn:

is a superficial burn; only the top layer of the skin is damaged.

You may see:

◆ reddened, dry skin, slight swelling

The casualty may complain of:

◆ pain ranging from mild to severe

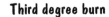

First degree burn

Second degree burn:

is a partial thickness burn; the second layer and the top layer are damaged

You may see:

◆ raw, moist skin, from white to cherry red, blisters with weeping clear fluid

The casualty may complain of:

◆ extreme pain

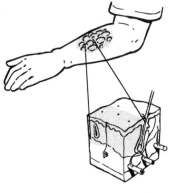

Second degree burn

Third degree burn:

is a deep burn with the full thickness of the skin destroyed; damage may also extend into the underlaying layers of nerves, muscles and fatty tissue. Third degree burns are often accompanied by very painful second degree burns.

You may see:

◆ white, waxy skin, becoming dry and leathery
◆ charred skin and underlaying tissues

The casualty may complain of:

◆ very little or no pain in the deeply burned area

Third degree burn

7

Mark each statement below as true **(T)** or false **(F)**.

☐ A. A casualty with a burn covering the surface of the forearm may suffer severe pain.

☐ B. Burns are classified according to the amount of skin surface burned.

☐ C. In a first degree burn the skin will show many blisters.

☐ D. Where the burn is very deep and the nerves are damaged, the casualty may not feel any pain.

☐ E. Blackened skin layers indicate a deep burn.

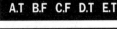
A.T B.F C.F D.T E.T

Seriousness of a burn

8

The seriousness of a burn depends on the:

◆ degree or depth of the burn
◆ amount of body surface burned

This can be determined by the **rule of nines** by dividing the body into multiples of nine. The larger the surface burned, the more serious is the burn.

◆ location of the burn
◆ age of the casualty

Medical help is always required when the burn:

◆ is deep
◆ covers a large area
◆ is located on the face, mouth or throat and can interfere with breathing
◆ is caused by chemicals or an electric current
◆ involves an infant or elderly person

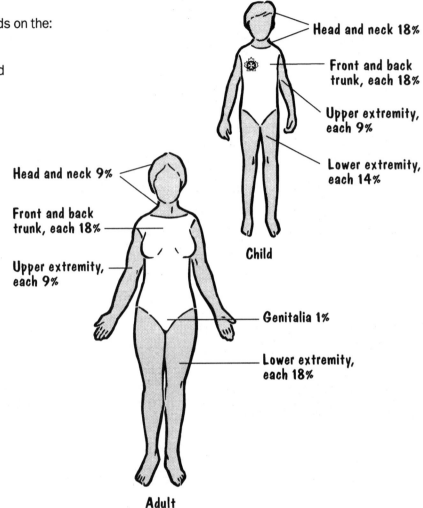

Head and neck 18%
Front and back trunk, each 18%
Upper extremity, each 9%
Lower extremity, each 14%
Child

Head and neck 9%
Front and back trunk, each 18%
Upper extremity, each 9%
Genitalia 1%
Lower extremity, each 18%
Adult

9

Which of the burn casualties described below would require immediate medical help?

Check ☑ the correct answers.

☐ A. A man splashes acid on his arms, neck and chest.
☐ B. A ten month old baby spilled boiling water over both his arms.
☐ C. A woman burns her hand on a hot kitchen stove.
☐ D. An 80-year old man burns his thigh and arm on a wood stove.
☐ E. After sunbathing a young girl has reddish skin on her back that is slightly swollen and painful.
☐ F. A teenager has difficulties swallowing after gulping down a cup of steaming hot tea.

A B D F

Smoke inhalation

10

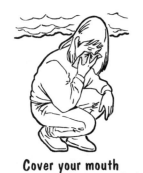

Cover your mouth and nose with a wet cloth

The air passages and the lungs can be seriously damaged by inhaling smoke from a fire.

To reduce the risk of smoke inhalation:

◆ stay close to the ground

◆ cover your mouth and nose with a wet cloth

◆ get out of the area as quickly as possible

◆ in industrial fires, don't enter the fire area without the proper safety equipment

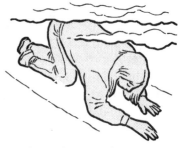

Stay close to the ground

If your clothing catches fire:

◆ **STOP** moving—don't run

◆ **DROP** to the ground

◆ **ROLL** several times to put the flames out

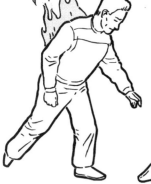

STOP

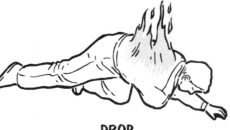

DROP

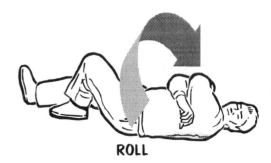

ROLL

11

You are trying to escape from of a room engulfed in flames. Your jacket has started to burn. Which of the following actions should you take to prevent serious burn damage to yourself?

From the options below, check ☑ the correct answers.

◻ A. Roll on the floor if your clothes are on fire.

◻ B. Get up and run towards the door.

◻ C. Crawl on the floor towards the door.

◻ D. Breath through a moist handkerchief.

◻ E. Open the windows for more fresh air.

A C D

First aid for heat burns

12

When you get burned, **immediately cool the burned area:**

◆ immerse the burned part in **cool water** until pain is relieved
◆ remove jewellery
◆ loosen tight clothing before swelling occurs

If immersing the burned area is not possible, you should:

◆ gently pour cool water over the burned area or
◆ apply a clean cloth soaked in cool water

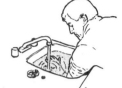

Immerse in cool water

Cooling a burn will:

◆ **reduce** the temperature of the burned area and prevent further tissue damage
◆ **reduce** swelling and blistering
◆ **relieve** pain

When the pain has lessened:

◆ cover the burned area loosely with a clean, preferably sterile material
◆ secure the dressing, ensuring that the tape does **not** touch the burned area.
◆ obtain medical help

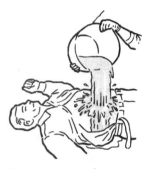

**Gently pour cool water
over the burned area**

or

13

Check ☑ the correct answer **to each of the following questions.**

You have just burned your hand on a hot stove. Which of the following actions should you do to relieve your pain and avoid more injury to the burned area?

☐ A. Soak your hand in a sink filled with lukewarm water.
☐ B. Cover the burned part with an adhesive dressing.
☐ C. Soak your hand in a sink filled with cool water.
☐ D. Take off any rings from your fingers.

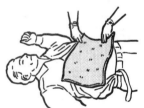

**Cover with wet,
cool cloth**

A man received a burn to his chest and stomach area. How should you lessen his pain while awaiting medical help?

☐ E. Rinse the affected area with cool, salted water.
☐ F. Apply direct pressure to the burned area.
☐ G. Cover the burn with cool, moist cloths.
☐ H. Apply towels soaked in warm water to the burn.

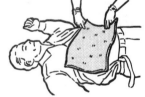

**Cover with clean
material**

C D G

First aid for chemical burns

14

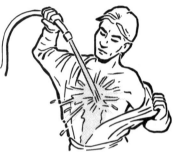

A **corrosive chemical** will continue to burn as long as it is in contact with the skin. To minimize the damage from corrosive chemicals on the skin, **speed is essential**:

- begin scene survey
- **immediately flush the area** with **cool** water
- if necessary, perform a primary survey and give first aid for life-threatening conditions
- flush during removal of clothing
- flush the area **for 15 to 20 minutes**

Remove clothing while flushing

If the corrosive chemical is a **dry powder**:

- remove contaminated clothing
- brush off any dry powder from the skin
  - ❖ **do not use your bare hands!**
- flush the affected area with cool water **for 15 to 20 minutes**

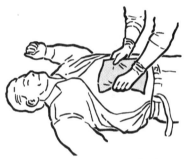

Following flushing:

- cover the burned area with a clean dressing
- obtain medical help

Cover burned area with clean material

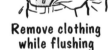

Remove clothing while flushing

Note: First aid for specific burns, e.g. from liquid sulphur, may vary from these general rules. You should know the chemicals used in your workplace and the recommended first aid.

15

A workman has spilled a strong corrosive liquid on his arms and chest. What action should he take **first**?

From the following options, check ☑ the correct answer.

- ☐ A. Cover the affected area with clean, moist dressings and obtain medical help.
- ☐ B. Remove his shirt and pants, and then pour water over the body.
- ☐ C. Flush his upper body with cool water while taking off his shirt and pants and continue flooding for about 15 minutes.
- ☐ D. Take off his shirt and pants first, then pour buckets of warm water over his body for about 5 minutes.

C

First aid for electrical burns

. . . .

16

Burns from an electric current may be more serious than they appear. As well as deep, **third degree** burns at the point of entry and exit, an electric shock can also cause:

◆ **stopped breathing**

◆ **cardiac arrest**

◆ **fractures and dislocations**

To give first aid:

◆ begin scene survey

◆ shut off the current, **or**
get the casualty away from the electrical source, if safe to do so

◆ perform primary survey and give life-saving first aid

  ❖ check for breathing and give AR if needed

  ❖ check circulation and give CPR if there is no pulse

◆ cover the entry and exit wounds with clean dry dressings

◆ steady and support fractures and/or dislocations

◆ obtain medical help

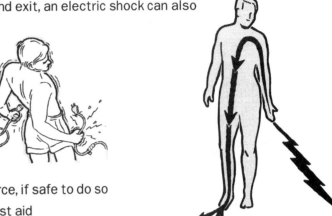

Electric current

Warning: Never approach a casualty of an electrical injury until the power is turned off. If there are downed wires, call for the power company or other officials to make the scene safe.

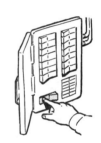

**Shut off the power
at the source**

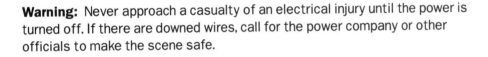

17

Mark each of the following statements as true **(T)** or false **(F)**.

☐ A. There will usually be only one deep wound from an electrical burn.

☐ B. When treating a casualty for burns from electricity, the burned areas are the top priority for first aid.

☐ C. A casualty's breathing and heart may stop following an electrical charge through his body.

☐ D. In an electrical incident, you should first drag the casualty from the source of electricity.

☐ E. When a casualty has received a violent electrical shock, you should suspect injuries to bones and joints.

A.F B.F C.T D.F E.T

First aid for radiation burns

18

Radioactive material burn

There is no specific first aid for radiation burns caused by radioactive materials. Workers involved with radioactive materials should learn the specific procedures and first aid for radioactive exposure. But first aid can be given for a radiation burn caused by the sun.

Minor sunburn

◆ Sponge the burned area with cool water
or cover the area with a cloth soaked in cool water

◆ Apply sunburn ointment or cream according to the direction on the label

   Caution: Some of these preparations may cause allergic reactions. Sunburn is the only burn to which an ointment is applied.

◆ Protect burned areas from the sun

◆ Do not break blisters

Major sunburn

◆ Give first aid as for heat burns

◆ If the casualty vomits or develops a fever get medical help immediately

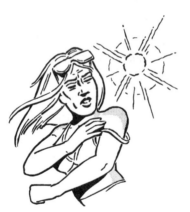

Minor sunburn

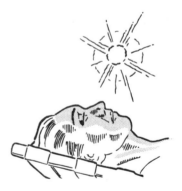

Major sunburn

19

From the statements below, check ☑ the correct first aid for a radiation burn.

☐ A. Towels drenched in cool water are soothing when applied to sunburned skin.

☐ B. Blisters caused by a sunburn should be drained before applying wet towels.

☐ C. Persons with a sunburn should be asked to stay in the shade.

☐ D. People who have been exposed to radioactive materials should get medical help.

☐ E. Creams sold to treat a sunburn can be safely used by everyone.

A C D

Complications that may result from burns

20

A burn may be complicated by:

◆ **breathing problems**
  ❖ severe burns about the face indicate the casualty may have inhaled hot smoke or fumes

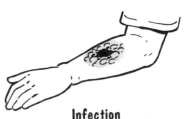

Infection

◆ **shock**
  ❖ caused by loss of body fluids and pain

◆ **infection**
  ❖ is a serious threat when the skin is burned and underlying tissue is exposed

◆ **swelling**
  ❖ particularly if jewellery or tight clothing cuts off circulation to the burned area

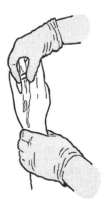

Precautions when giving first aid for burns

When giving first aid for a burn, avoid causing further injury and contamination.

◆ **DO NOT** overcool the casualty causing a dangerous lowering of body temperature
◆ **DO NOT** remove anything sticking to the burn. This may cause further damage and contamination

Take off rings before swelling occurs

◆ **DO NOT** break blisters
◆ **DO NOT** touch the burn with your fingers
◆ **DO NOT** breathe, talk or cough over the burn
◆ **DO NOT** apply lotions, oils, butter or fat to the injury
◆ **DO NOT** cover the burn with cotton wool, adhesive dressings or tape

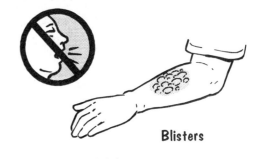

Blisters

21

Mark each statement below that describes how to prevent complications of burns as true **(T)** or false **(F)**.

☐ A. Watch for breathing difficulties of the burned casualty.
☐ B. Watch for signs of pale, cold, clammy skin and a weak, rapid pulse.
☐ C. Remove any rings before the tissue swells.
☐ D. Pull away a casualty's blouse that is clinging to the burned skin.
☐ E. Use your clean fingers to remove pieces of burned skin and clothing.
☐ F. Drain blisters before applying a dressing.

A.T B.T C.T D.F E.F F.F

Objectives

• •

Following the video and upon completion of this activity book exercise, in an emergency situation, you will be able to:

◆ take measures to prevent burns

◆ recognize burns

◆ provide first aid for burns

For further information on burns, please refer to:
First on the Scene, the St. John Ambulance first aid and CPR manual, chapter 9, available through your instructor or any major bookstore in your area.

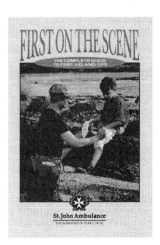

EXERCISE 21

MEDICAL CONDITIONS

(DIABETES, CONVULSIONS, ASTHMA & ALLERGIES)

Diabetic emergencies

1

The body needs **energy** to function. The energy comes from sugar that the body gets from the food you eat.

Diabetes is a condition in which the body cannot convert sugar into energy because of **a lack of insulin**.

Insulin is a substance produced by the body to regulate the use of sugar. Normally there is a balance between the sugar used and the insulin produced.

A **diabetic emergency** occurs when there is a severe imbalance between the amount of insulin and sugar in the body.

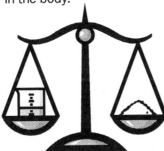

Normal balance between insulin and sugar

2

Mark each of the following statements as either true **(T)** or false **(F)**.

- [ ] A. Sugar acts as a fuel for the body.
- [ ] B. Insulin is supplied to the body by way of the food we eat.
- [ ] C. Insulin controls the sugar level in the body.
- [ ] D. A person who has diabetes has a sugar imbalance because of a lack of insulin.

A.T   B.F   C.T   D.T

3

Causes of diabetic emergencies

Diabetes is a condition in which the body does **not produce enough insulin,** causing the sugar level to be out of balance.

To balance the sugar level, a person with diabetes may take prescribed amounts of the medication, either by mouth or by injection.

Two conditions may result in a diabetic emergency:

Not enough insulin, causing a high level of sugar—diabetic coma (also called hyperglycemia)

Too much insulin, causing a low level of sugar—insulin shock (also called hypoglycemia)

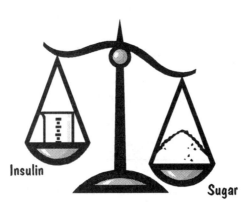

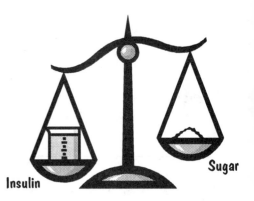

May be caused by:

◆ not taking enough insulin

◆ eating too much food

◆ doing less exercise than usual

May be caused by:

◆ taking too much insulin

◆ not eating enough food or vomiting

◆ doing more exercise than usual

4

Which of the following situations may lead to a diabetic emergency?

Check ☑ the correct answers.

☐ A. A diabetic person has regular insulin shots and watches his diet and exercise.

☐ B. An elderly non-diabetic person loves to eat sweets.

☐ C. A diabetic person misses dinner.

☐ D. A man forgets to take his prescribed amount of insulin.

☐ E. A young diabetic person competes in an unscheduled bicycle race.

How to recognize a diabetic emergency

5

A **conscious casualty with diabetes** might be able to tell you what is wrong. However, keep in mind that the person may be confused.

An **unconscious casualty** may be wearing a **medical alert** bracelet or necklace that will tell you that she has diabetes.

If the casualty cannot tell you what she needs, look for the following signs and symptoms:

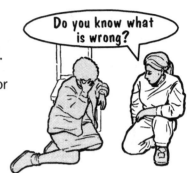

	Insulin shock (needs sugar)	Diabetic coma (needs insulin)
Pulse:	strong and rapid	weak and rapid
Breathing:	shallow	deep and sighing
Skin:	pale and sweating	flushed, dry and warm
Breath odour:	odourless	like musty apple or nail polish
LOC:	faintness to unconsciousness developing quickly	gradual onset of unconsciousness
Other signs and symptoms	headache trembling hunger	unsteady walk nausea

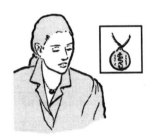

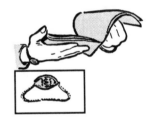

Medical alert devices

6

Which of the following actions will help you to assess the casualty's condition as a diabetic emergency?

Check ☑ the correct answers.

- ☐ A. Ask the conscious casualty about her condition.
- ☐ B. Look for some information on the unconscious casualty that identifies her as having diabetes.
- ☐ C. Keep asking the casualty questions, even if the response does not make sense.
- ☐ D. When the conscious casualty tells you that she has diabetes, ask whether she has had her normal food and insulin that day.

A B D

First aid for a diabetic emergency

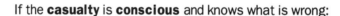

7

The first aid for insulin shock and diabetic coma is the same:

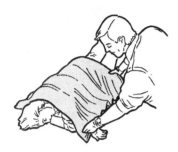

Unresponsive casualty

- begin scene survey
  - ❖ if the casualty is **unresponsive**, get medical help immediately
- do a primary survey and give first aid for life-threatening conditions
- place the unconscious person into the recovery position and monitor the ABCs until medical help takes over
- look for a medical alert device that will give you more information about the casualty's condition

If the **casualty** is **conscious** and knows what is wrong:

- assist her to take what is needed—**sugar or her prescribed medication**

If the casualty is **confused** about what is required:

- give her something sweet to eat or drink and get medical help

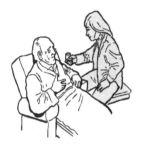

Give something sweet

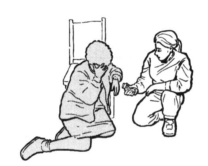

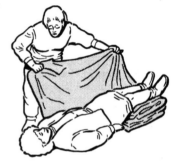

Shock position

8

Which of the following actions should you take when a diabetic emergency occurs?

Check ☑ the correct answers.

- ☐ A. Give a conscious diabetic person several glasses of cool water to drink.
- ☐ B. Give a conscious casualty candy or orange juice if she is not sure what she needs.
- ☐ C. Send someone to telephone for medical help if the sweetened drink does not improve the casualty's condition.
- ☐ D. Place an unconscious diabetic person in the best position to ensure an open airway.
- ☐ E. Help a conscious casualty to take her medication if she says she needs it and asks for your assistance.

How to recognize an epileptic seizure

. . . .

9

Epilepsy is a disorder of the nervous system. It may result in recurring convulsions, called **epileptic seizures,** involving partial or complete loss of consciousness. In most cases epilepsy is controlled by medication and seizures don't happen often. An **epileptic seizure** may come on **suddenly** and **be very brief.**

Any of the following signs and symptoms will help you to identify a major epileptic seizure–

You may see:

◆ the casualty falling to the floor
◆ sudden loss of consciousness
◆ noisy breathing
◆ frothing at the mouth
◆ grinding of teeth
◆ convulsions (uncontrollable muscle contractions) with arching of the back
◆ the casualty may loose control over bladder and bowel functions

Some casualties may complain of:

◆ a sensation such as a sound, smell or feeling of movement in the body that tells them that a seizure is about to occur. This is called an **aura.**

On regaining consciousness the person may be unaware of recent events and be confused and very tired.

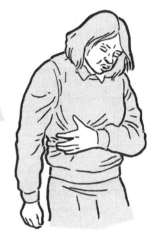

Aura

. . . .

10

Mark each of the following statements as either true **(T)** or false **(F).**

☐ A. A person with epilepsy always experiences a feeling that convulsions are about to happen.

☐ B. Epileptic seizures are usually of short duration and may occur at any time.

☐ C. A person who has passed out during the seizure may not remember the incident on recovery.

☐ D. A person's mouth is usually dry and hangs open during an epileptic seizure.

☐ E. During a seizure, the person has no control over his movements and may gasp for air.

First aid for an epileptic seizure

11

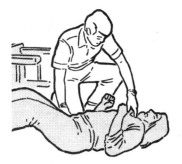

Make area safe

The **aim of first aid** for an epileptic seizure is to protect the casualty from injury during the period of convulsions.

You should:

◆ begin scene survey
◆ clear the area of hard or sharp objects that could cause injury
◆ clear the area of onlookers to **ensure privacy** for the casualty
◆ **guide** but **do not restrict** movement
◆ carefully loosen tight clothing
◆ turn the casualty gently to the side with the face turned slightly downward. This will allow for drainage and prevent her tongue from falling back into her throat
◆ **do not** attempt to force the casualty's mouth open or to put anything between her teeth

When convulsions have stopped:

◆ place her into the recovery position and wipe away any fluids from the mouth and nose
◆ do a secondary survey to see if the casualty was injured during the seizure
◆ give ongoing casualty care, monitor breathing and allow her to rest

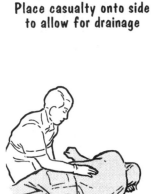

Place casualty onto side to allow for drainage

The casualty usually recovers quickly. If you know the convulsions were caused by epilepsy, you do not need to call medical help.

Call for medical help:

◆ if a second seizure occurs within minutes
◆ if the casualty is unconscious for more than five minutes
◆ if it is the person's first seizure or the cause is unknown

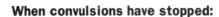

12

Recovery position

A woman in a crowded store suddenly falls to the floor and goes into convulsions. What should you do?

Check ☑ the correct answers.

- [ ] A. Tell the bystanders to form a circle around the woman.
- [ ] B. Clear away all objects on which she could hurt herself.
- [ ] C. Hold her arms firmly to prevent injury.
- [ ] D. Watch her closely to ensure she is breathing.
- [ ] E. Position her to maintain an open airway.

B D E

Convulsions in children

. . . .

13

An infant or young child with a **rapid rise in body temperature** to 40°C or 104°F is at risk of convulsions. A fever emergency is when the temperature taken in the armpit is 38°C (100.5°F) or higher for an infant and 40°C (104°F) or higher for a child.

First aid for fever may prevent the onset of convulsions

Advise the parent/caregiver to:

◆ call the doctor immediately and follow her advice

◆ give acetaminophen (e.g. Tempra® or Tylenol® according to directions on the label)if the doctor can't be reached

◆ **not give ASA** (e.g. Aspirin®), it may cause Reye's syndrome, a life-threatening condition, in children and adolescents

◆ encourage the child to drink fluids

◆ sponge the child with lukewarm water for about 20 minutes if the temperature doesn't go down. Don't immerse the child in a tub

◆ monitor the child's temperature and repeat these steps if necessary

Fever convulsions can be recognized by the same signs as an epileptic seizure (see page 21–5).

First aid for fever convulsions is to:

◆ protect the child from injury. Clear the area of hard or sharp objects that could cause injury

◆ loosen constrictive clothing

◆ not restrain the child

When convulsions cease:

◆ place the child into the best recovery position for his age, with the head lowered and turned to one side

◆ reassure the child's parents

◆ obtain medical help

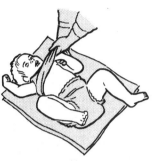

Remove clothing

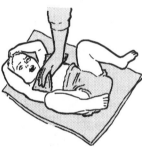

Sponge with tepid water

. . . .

14

Which of the following actions should you take when a two-year old child is having high fever and convulsions? Check ☑ the correct answers.

To bring down the fever:

☐ A. Follow the doctor's advice.

During convulsions:

☐ B. Hold her arms and legs tightly so she won't hurt herself.

☐ C. Unbutton her shirt at the neck.

☐ D. Ensure that she is breathing effectively.

When the convulsions have stopped:

☐ E. Position her flat on her back.

☐ F. Tell her parent to try not to worry.

A C D F

Asthma

. . . .

15

Bronchial asthma, often simply called, **asthma,** involves repeated attacks of shortness of breath with wheezing and coughing.

Asthma causes narrowing of the airways in the lungs which is due to:

◆ tightening of the muscles in the airways

◆ swelling of the inner lining of the airway (bronchi and bronchioles)

◆ an increase in the amount and thickness of the mucus

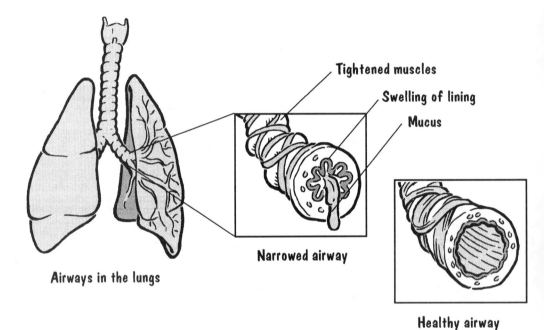

Airways in the lungs

Tightened muscles

Swelling of lining

Mucus

Narrowed airway

Healthy airway

. . . .

16

Check ☑ the statements below which correctly explain why the airways narrow.

☐ A. The lining of the airways becomes thicker.

☐ B. The mucus becomes thinner and more scanty.

☐ C. The muscles in the walls of the airways contract.

☐ D. More mucus develops and it becomes stickier.

Causes of an acute asthmatic attack

· ·

17

Asthmatic attacks are usually caused by exposure to certain **triggers.** These triggers vary widely among people with asthma.

Common triggers include, e.g.:

◆ house dust
◆ smoke
◆ pollen
◆ insects
◆ furry or feathered animals, e.g. dogs, cats, birds
◆ certain foods
◆ certain drugs
◆ a cold
◆ stress/emotional upsets

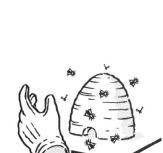

Although asthmatic attacks can be triggered unexpectedly, preventive measures can be taken by avoiding triggers known to cause an attack.

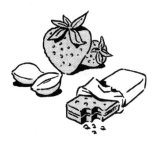 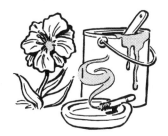 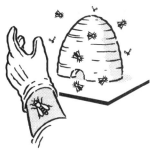

Triggers for allergic reaction/asthma

· ·

18

Check ☑ the correct statements below which indicate how you could help prevent certain triggers to cause an asthmatic attack.

☐ A. Regularly clean floors with a damp mop.
☐ B. Don't use rugs or drapes which collect dust.
☐ C. Avoid disturbing stinging insects.
☐ D. Allow your kitten to sleep on your bed.
☐ E. Use a down-filled quilt for warmth in the winter.
☐ F. Avoid grasses or flowers which have caused breathing problems for you in the past.

A B C F

How to recognize a severe asthmatic attack

. . . .

19

Asthmatic attacks vary in how rapidly they begin, how severe they are and how long they last. A **mild** asthmatic attack can be annoying. A **severe** asthmatic attack can be fatal.

You can recognize a **severe asthmatic attack** by the following signs and symptoms:

- shortness of breath with obvious trouble breathing
- coughing or wheezing (a whistling noise when air moves through the narrowed airways) may get louder or stop
- fast and shallow breathing
- tightness in the chest
- casualty sitting upright trying to breathe
- bluish colour in the face
- fast pulse rate
- anxiety
- restlessness, then fatigue
- shock

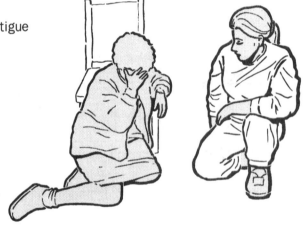

. . . .

20

Mark each of the following statements as either true **(T)** or false **(F)**.

- [ ] A. Shortness of breath eases as an asthmatic attack becomes more severe.
- [ ] B. All people with asthma wheeze during a severe asthmatic attack.
- [ ] C. Wheezing is the sound of air in smaller than normal airways.
- [ ] D. If a person with asthma is anxious, has sweaty, bluish/grey skin, is sitting and has difficulty with each breath, the attack is severe.

A.F B.F C.T D.T

First aid for a severe asthmatic attack

21

If the casualty shows increasing breathing difficulties:

You should:

◆ call for medical help immediately

◆ have the casualty stop any activity

◆ place the casualty in the most comfortable position for breathing.
This is usually sitting upright, leaning slightly forward and resting on a support

◆ provide reassurance because fear will increase the breathing rate

◆ do not encourage drinking during an attack. Fluids may get into the lungs

◆ assist the casualty to take her prescribed medication if you are asked to do so (see next page)

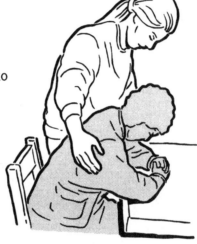

Position casualty

22

A middle aged man shows signs of a severe asthmatic attack with more and more trouble breathing. To help him, which choice of action should you take?

Check ☑ your choices.

Choice 1

☐ A. Call for an ambulance as soon as possible.

☐ B. Lay the casualty down to rest.

☐ C. Give plenty of fluids to loosen the mucus.

☐ D. Calm the casualty to relieve anxiety.

Choice 2

☐ A. Call for an ambulance when the casualty stops breathing.

☐ B. Have the man sit up to make breathing easier.

☐ C. Don't let the man have anything to drink.

☐ D. Encourage the man to breathe faster.

A.1 B.2 C.2 D.1

Assisting with inhalers

. . . .

23

The casualty may be too weak or is breathing too rapidly to use the inhaler herself. You can assist the casualty to take her prescribed medication as follows:

Inhaler with collecting chamber and mask

1

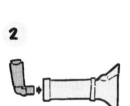

- ◆ the casualty must **ask for your assistance** and indicate clearly which medication is to be used
- ◆ ask for a nod as an answer to your questions to save the casualty from speaking
- ◆ ask if the container needs to be shaken and assist if needed
- ◆ remove the cap and hand the inhaler to the casualty for her to use
  - ❖ it is not unusual for an asthmatic to take 5 to 10 puffs
- ◆ if assisting with inhalers is not possible, monitor breathing closely
- ◆ provide ongoing casualty care until medical help takes over

2

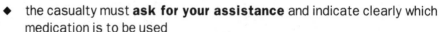

1

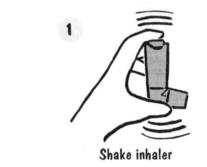

Shake inhaler

3

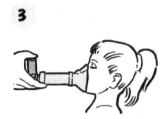

2

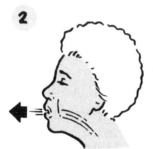

3

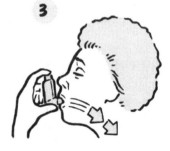

. . . .

24

Mark each of the following statements as either true **(T)** or false **(F)**.

- ☐ A. You should give medication for asthmatic attacks immediately when you see that a person has problems breathing.
- ☐ B. Not all inhalers require shaking before use.
- ☐ C. If the casualty cannot speak, you should immediately give her the prescribed medication.
- ☐ D. Several puffs of medication may be required to relieve the breathing difficulties.

Allergic reactions

. . . .

25

An **allergic reaction** is the response of a body with an abnormal sensitivity to substances that are normally harmless.

Substances causing allergic reactions **enter the body by**:

◆ swallowing (e.g. foods, medications)

◆ inhaling (e.g. dust, pollen)

◆ absorption through the skin (e.g. plants, chemicals)

◆ injection (bee/wasp stings, drugs)

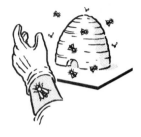

The severity of an allergic reaction varies from minor discomfort to a **severe life-threatening type of shock** (anaphylactic shock).

You can recognize a severe allergic reaction by any of the following:

You may see:

◆ sneezing, coughing and red watery eyes

◆ swelling of the face, mouth and throat

◆ laboured breathing with wheezing due to swollen tissues obstructing the airway

◆ a weak, rapid pulse

◆ vomiting and diarrhea

◆ pale skin, blueness or both

◆ changes in level of consciousness

The casualty may complain of:

◆ tightness in the chest

◆ severe itching with hives (raised skin eruptions)

◆ dizziness

◆ abdominal cramps with nausea

An asthmatic attack is an allergic reaction that results in breathing problems.

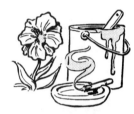

Triggers

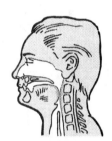

Inflamed airway
passages

. . . .

26

Which of the following observations may help you to recognize an allergic reaction? Check ☑ the correct answers.

☐ A. Smooth, pale skin on the body.

☐ B. Difficult breathing.

☐ C. Violent shivering.

☐ D. Puffy face and irritations of the skin.

☐ E. Indigestion and a loose bowel movement.

☐ F. Unsteadiness.

B D E F

First aid for severe allergic reactions

EpiPen® Auto-Injector **27**

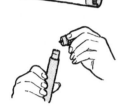

A person who has a known, severe allergy, usually carries this information on him:

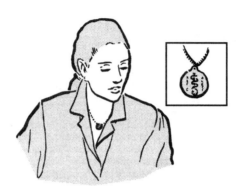

Medical alert
necklace

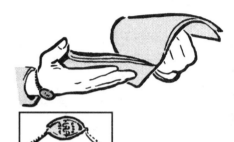

Medical alert bracelet

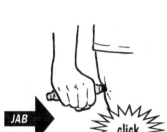

JAB click

Ana-Kit®

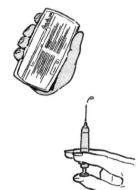

Give **first aid** as follows:

◆ send for medical help
◆ monitor airway, breathing, circulation (ABC's)
◆ maintain breathing and circulation
◆ check for medical alert information
◆ assist the conscious casualty to take prescribed medication, e.g. Ana-Kit® or EpiPen® Auto Injector. Follow the casualty's instructions and the manufacturer's directions. The medication will begin to wear off within 10 to 20 minutes
◆ provide care for shock until medical help takes over

Watch the casualty carefully. An allergic reaction can become life-threatening.

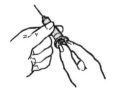

28

Check ☑ the procedures you would follow to give first aid to a person who is having a severe allergic reaction.

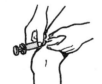

☐ A. Call for medical assistance immediately when you note signs of shock.
☐ B. If the casualty has an allergy kit, take him and the kit to a doctor.
☐ C. Ensure adequate breathing and provide artificial respiration if required.
☐ D. Monitor the person's condition continuously until medical personnel takes over or the person has fully recovered.

A C D

Medical conditions—review

· ·

29

1. You have a casualty who has asthma and is wheezing noisily. Which illustration below shows the best position for this condition? Check ☑ the correct answer.

☐ A.
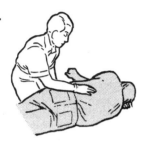

☐ B.
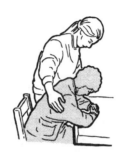

2. Which two illustrations below show the correct first aid for a diabetic casualty who has not eaten for a long time and is feeling sick? Check ☑ the correct answers.

☐ A. Help with an inhaler.

☐ B. Give something sweet.

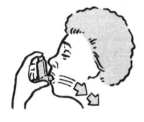

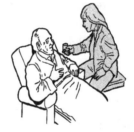

☐ C. Turn into the recovery position.

☐ D. Call for medical help.

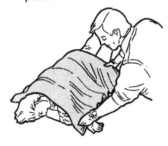

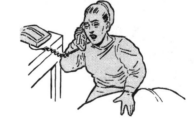

☐ E. Help with an allergy injection.

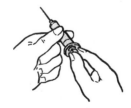

Objectives

● ●

Upon completion of this activity book exercise, in an emergency situation, you will be able to:

◆ recognize a diabetic emergency

◆ provide first aid for a diabetic emergency

◆ recognize an epileptic seizure

◆ provide first aid for an epileptic seizure

◆ recognize convulsions in children

◆ provide first aid for convulsions in children

◆ recognize a severe asthma attack and provide first aid

◆ recognize a severe allergic reaction and provide first aid

For further information on medical conditions, please refer to:
First on the Scene, the St. John Ambulance first aid and CPR manual, chapter 11, available through your instructor or any major bookstore in your area.

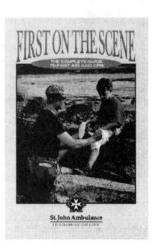

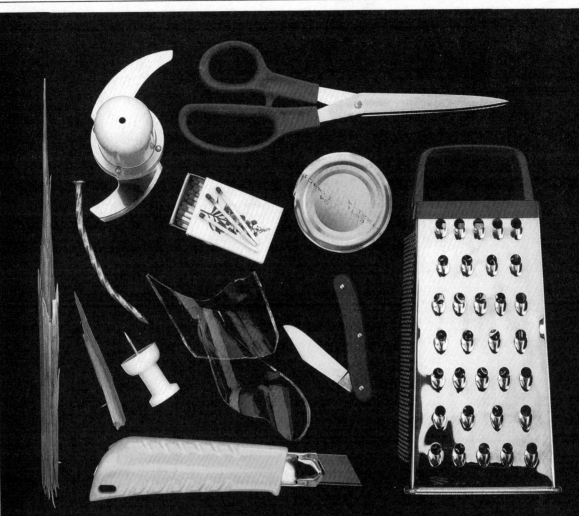

The reasons for buying our Family First Aid Kit are painfully obvious.

Family life is filled with cuts, scrapes and scratches. Some can be serious. The St. John Ambulance Family First Aid Kit provides you with first aid for all types of injuries. It's like a security blanket for the whole family. So order yours today. Being without one could prove to be a pain.

For details about this or other St. John Ambulance First Aid Kits ask your instructor or contact your local branch.

St. John Ambulance

WHAT NEXT?!

Congratulations!

You have successfully completed a St. John Ambulance First Aid course. What next? Why not put your new skills to use, and become a volunteer member of St. John Ambulance.

Join the Brigade

▶ **serve your community**—provide first aid services at local events, and take part in other programmes such as hospital or school visits.

▶ **learn more first aid, CPR and patient care skills (free of charge)**—ongoing training for Brigade members integrates first aid, CPR and patient care skills along with practical and written assessments.

▶ **develop leadership skills**—take advantage of leadership training and apply it in leadership positions at all levels of the Brigade.

▶ **make new friends**—there are approximately 500 Brigade divisions across the country, made up of over 11,000 people, like yourself, who want to share their time and skills with their communities.

▶ **earn recognition**—your involvement in the Brigade will be appreciated by employers and schools. Your achievements will be recognized through our extensive awards programme.

Become an Instructor

▶ **teach courses to the public**—further your knowledge and techniques through the National Instructor Training and Development Programme, and share your talents through community-based courses.

▶ **earn an honorarium**—expenses incurred by you in implementing courses will be covered by an honorarium.

▶ **help Canadians to help themselves**—with your help, Canadians will learn new skills in the variety of courses offered by St. John Ambulance.

▶ **gain experience speaking in front of a group**—you will have an opportunity to speak to Canadians young and old, and from a variety of cultural backgrounds. Each new group offers new and different challenges.

▶ **develop lasting friendships**—participating as a St. John instructor will have a positive effect on you not only from fellow instructors but also from your students.

Share your skills—join the St. John family.
For more information, contact your
local Branch of St. John Ambulance today!

St. John Ambulance

Answers to the instructor-led exercises

· ·

For your reference, the answers to the instructor-led exercises throughout the work-
book are given below:

Instructor-led Exercise 4

A1 can

A2 forceful

A3 wheezing

A4 reddish

A5 encourage coughing

B1 cannot

B2 ineffective

B3 high-pitched noises

B4 bluish

B5 first aid

C1 cannot

C2 impossible

C3 no sound; cannot

C4 bluish

C5 first aid

Instructor-led Exercise 8A

1. blood pressure

2. constantly

3a. thick and less elastic

b. enlarged

4. almost never

5. fatty deposits

6. b

7. coronary artery disease

8. a, b, c, d, f

9. oxygen

10. narrowed

11. blood clot; heart muscle

12. oxygen

13. angina

14. pumping blood

15. sudden death

16. (in any order)

heart attack

stroke

electrical shock

poisoning

suffocation

drowning

17. oxygen

18. blockage; brain

19. stroke

Instructor-led Exercise 8B

Angina/Heart attack

A1 do it's work without pain

A2 heart tissue alive

A3 chest

A4 spread

A5 denial; vomiting

A6 scene survey

A7 primary survey

A8 send or go

A10 conscious

A11 medical help takes over

Cardiac arrest

B1 stopped beating; pumping

B3 breathing

B4 pulse

B5 scene survey

B6 responsiveness

B7 send or go

B8 CPR

Stroke/TIA

C1 brain; dies

C2 does not die

C3 changes

C4 pupils

C5 speak

C6 paralyzed

C9 TIA

C10 scene survey

C11 primary survey

C12 send or go

C13 comfortable; loosen

C14 nothing

C15 protect

C16 the recovery position;
paralyzed

C17 medical help takes over

FIRST AID—EMERGENCY LEVEL
Student course evaluation

Today's date _____

Instructor's name _____

Your opinion is valuable to us!

Please complete this course evaluation—your answers will help us to serve you and others better! Your answers will remain confidential.

1. What were your top three reasons for taking a first aid course? Place a check mark ☑ beside your reasons in the order of importance to you. Check only three.

Rank			Reason
1st	2nd	3rd	
—	—	—	Job requirement
—	—	—	Educational requirement
—	—	—	Because of a family member's health
—	—	—	Personal interest
—	—	—	Skill desired as a new parent
—	—	—	Other (specify)_____

2. When was your last first aid course? (check ☑ one)
   ☐ never ☐ less than 3 yrs ☐ more than 3 yrs

3. **Quality of the Course Components**
   Circle N/A if a course component was not used (e.g. videos).

   Rate specific points for each of the following, where "1" is not at all and "5" is very much.

Activity book	Not at all		N/A		Very much
informative	1	2	3	4	5
easy to understand	1	2	3	4	5
illustrations helpful	1	2	3	4	5
questions helpful	1	2	3	4	5

Comments:
_____
_____
_____
_____
_____

Practical exercises	Not at all		N/A		Very much
well organized	1	2	3	4	5
enough time to practise	1	2	3	4	5
increased your confidence	1	2	3	4	5

Comments:
_____
_____
_____
_____
_____

Video	Not at all		N/A		Very much
presented first aid					
skills clearly	1	2	3	4	5
helped you to learn	1	2	3	4	5

Comments:
_____
_____
_____
_____

Exam	Not at all		N/A		Very much
questions were clear	1	2	3	4	5
based on what you learned	1	2	3	4	5
enough time to complete	1	2	3	4	5
instructor reviewed answers	1	2	3	4	5
exam booklet and answer sheet					
were easy to use together	1	2	3	4	5

Comments:
_____
_____
_____
_____

Quality of Instruction

	Not at all			Very much	
informative lectures	1	2	3	4	5
clear demonstrations	1	2	3	4	5
knowledgeable instructor	1	2	3	4	5
effective use of time	1	2	3	4	5
efficient class administration	1	2	3	4	5

Comments:

_____

_____

_____

_____

_____

_____

Overall Course

	Not at all			Very much	
How well did the course meet your expectations/needs?	1	2	3	4	5

Would you take another
St. John Ambulance course? ☐ yes ☐ no

	Not at all			Very much	
How prepared do you feel to give first aid in an emergency?	1	2	3	4	5

Comments:

_____

_____

_____

_____

_____

_____

4. Please check ☑ the appropriate boxes below.

a. Language(s) spoken at home:
   ☐ English
   ☐ French
   ☐ Other (specify) _____

b. Gender   ☐ Female   ☐ Male

c. Age Group

☐ 10 – 13	☐ 35 – 44
☐ 14 – 15	☐ 45 – 54
☐ 16 – 19	☐ 55 – 69
☐ 20 – 24	☐ 70 and over
☐ 25 – 34	

5. Circle the highest level of education completed.
   ☐ Elementary
   ☐ Secondary
   ☐ Community College
   ☐ University

6. Other comments:

_____

_____

_____

_____

_____

This course was taken at:

Council

| NT ☐ | BC ☐ | AB ☐ | SK ☐ | MB ☐ | ON ☐ |
| QC ☐ | NS ☐ | NB ☐ | PE ☐ | NF ☐ | FD ☐ |

or

Special Centre

Air Canada ☐	Bell Canada ☐	Canada Post ☐
Canadian Airlines ☐	CN ☐	Fed Govt ☐
Canadian Pacific ☐	DND ☐	Eatons ☐
Northern Telecom ☐	RCMP ☐	VIA Rail ☐

Thank you for your help!